GET A GRIP
AND STAY SANE

GET A GRIP AND STAY SANE

Self-Healing
with the Nadi Technique

Billy Roberts

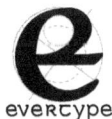

e
everτype
2016

Published by Evertype, 73 Woodgrove, Portlaoise, R32 ENP6, Ireland. *www.evertype.com*.

First edition 2016.

A catalogue record for this book is available from the British Library.

ISBN-10 1-78201-186-2
ISBN-13 978-1-78201-186-6

Typesetting by Michael Everson. Set in Baskerville and **Franklin Gothic**.

Cover design by Michael Everson. Abstract henna paisley-peacock background © Krishna Kharidehal.

Printed and bound by LightningSource.

Contents

INTRODUCTION

Introduction

Our parents are no doubt unwittingly the architects of our destinies, and from the earliest moments of our life on this planet our future is essentially in their hands. In fact, from a very early age our parents programme our minds and chastise us by imposing upon us their likes and dislikes, effectively creating us psychologically, emotionally and very often spiritually, in their own image, in very much the same way that their parents did to them, and so on through the family history. However, if we are fortunate enough to have well grounded, intelligent and far-seeing parents, then it's a fairly safe bet that you will do well in life, circumstances permitting, of course. However, there are other psychological factors to be considered; such as the impressions made on us by our peers and how much we are influenced by the people with whom we associate. We live to all intents and purposes in an extremely competitive world; and a world in which our human frailties and failings are constantly being put to the test, nearly always beyond our endurance. Little wonder then why many of us have lots of hang-ups, are insecure and lack confidence. We can't really help but admire those who have done well in life, occasionally to the extent of feeling somewhat jealous, or even resentful. "Good luck to them!" you may very well say, but if you're honest with yourself there is always a part of you that says, "I could have done better than that! If only..." There are many "If onlys" in everyone's life, and there is always a little jealousy when we see others achieve something that inwardly we know we could have done ten times better, given the opportunity that is. But that's just it, isn't it? The opportunity is never presented to those who don't expect it! But why do some people who appear to have no real talent get on in life and others with exceptional skills fail in everything they do? Or could it be that those who succeed in life resonate with some sort of universal magnetism that sets everything in motion for them, affording them success, good health, wealth and happiness? Or is success passed down to us from our forebears, through some sort of genetic electrical impulse system? I would say that there is far more to success than luck or good business acumen, and there is nearly always something a little special about those who succeed that makes them stand out from everyone else. They do say that if you desperately want to succeed in any chosen profession, to the extent that it preoccupies every aspect of your being, then the universe will always conspire to lead you into a position whereby your dreams and aspirations may successfully be gratified. Looking at it in this way then we are surely the architects of our own destinies, as long as, that is, we don't allow our parents' control of our minds to last forever, or to interfere with our dreams when we are young! However, as we do not have any say in the matter when we are children, we have to do what we are told, don't we? But in the majority of people there is the potential of a genius that lies dormant, waiting for that moment of arousal. For many that moment never arrives, simply because the dream is never really strong enough.

I was born into a working class family in Wavertree, a suburb of Liverpool, England, on 24 June 1946, at a time when the whole country was still recovering from the battering it had received from the German bombers in the so-called "Blitz" of the Second World War. Even though Liverpool, as well as other cities, had taken an incredible pounding, the camaraderie was incredible, and really did make the whole of the country a force to be reckoned with. When I was born, my mother and father,

INTRODUCTION

Annie and Albert Roberts already had a ten year old son, also called Albert (or Alby as he was and still is affectionately known), and so as far as they were concerned their family was complete. When I was three years old whooping cough left me with a serious respiratory disease called Bronchiectasis, (dilation of the bronchi) and as antibiotics were then in their embryonic stages, the prognosis for me was fairly bleak. My parents were told in no uncertain terms, that because the damage to my lungs was fairly extensive, I would most probably not live to see my 12 birthday. As a result of this I spent 20 weeks out of every year in Alder Hey Children's Hospital in Liverpool, England, and was mollycoddled and given everything I wanted by my parents. The very fact that they could not in any way see a future for me, had its psychological implications on my young life, making me insecure, introverted and extremely anxious, to the extent I hated being away from my mother. I became dependent on her for everything, and by the time I was five years old and had to go to school, I was a nervous wreck and, as a consequence, was perceived by other children with some amusement, as a "mummy's boy"! I learned at a very early age just how cruel other kids could be, and the more I was bullied the more I wanted so desperately to always be by myself. My mother constantly instilled in me that I was not at all like other children, and that I would never be able to achieve academic success. Although she may not have realized it, she was unwittingly conditioning my mind to become the person she herself believed I was. In fact, she was imposing psychological limitations on my development as a person, and in some way was making me believe that I would never be able to achieve a successful career in any profession. I suppose it came as somewhat of a surprise to my parents when I not only lived to see my twelfth birthday, but also my sixteenth, eighteenth, and so on. Of course, I wasn't academically qualified for anything, and because of my health I could not really do manual labour. I had always had a propensity for playing the guitar, and so my father bought me my very first electric guitar when I was twelve years old. By the time I left school in 1962 at the age of 16, I was already living the dream of every other kid my age—playing lead guitar in a Rock band and touring extensively. By the time I was 18 I had toured all over Europe supporting some of the biggest names in the music industry; from Chuck Berry and the Moody Blues, to Jimi Hendrix and the Yardbirds. Music was in fact all I'd ever wanted to do, and do it I did in more ways than one. Even though I played in large auditoriums as well as small venues, I was still very shy and insecure. In fact, I used to hide behind my guitar and didn't really want to be seen. As long as I could play music nothing else really mattered.

My band was then managed by Jean Vanlou, the director of Unidans, one of the largest agencies on the Continent. In fact, Jean Vanlou had been responsible for bringing Jimi Hendrix and many others to the Continent. He was an entrepreneur with an imposing personality, quietly spoken and a very gentle and kind man. We were resident at the Twenty Club in Mouscron, Belgium, owned by Jean Vanlou, and here we played most Sundays when we were not actually touring.

In between tours we had to return to the UK while our permits were renewed. In the UK during this time we played as many as 5 gigs a day, finishing off the day playing at a so-called "all-nighter" in Manchester and not getting back home until a little after 6am, totally exhausted. Although the other members of the band coped quite well, my overall health condition caused extreme fatigue with non-specific aches and pains. In the late 1950s my mother had been prescribed drynomol, commonly known as "Purple Hearts", an amphetamine based drug which she had been given to help her cope with the acute symptoms of the menopause. She always kept a large supply of these in brown bottles behind the clock on the sideboard in the living room. Seeing how exhausted I was, my mother gave me a handful and suggested I take them to give me a boost and whenever I needed to stay awake. Unknowingly she could not have done a worst thing. She was simply fuelling my inherent addictive nature and giving me a taste of something that was to eventually nearly cause my demise. My use of illicit substances escalated and by 1969 I returned to the UK, worn out and quite ill. I had a long battle ahead with very little help extended to me.

Of course, my use of cocaine and eventually heroin naturally impacted on the respiratory disease I'd lived with and managed for so many years. I began coughing copious amounts of blood (a symptom of bronchiectasis) and was so weak all I could do was sit in the armchair in front of the television in my mother's home day after day, until it was time to climb into bed at night. I knew I was dying and wanted it to come quickly. I eventually saw the glimmer of a light at the end of what had been a very long and dark and lonely tunnel, and I began to venture beyond the safety of my mother's home. Once away from the door, to my dread and horror, I found myself overwhelmed with panic. My legs felt like jelly, my heart began to race, the muscles across my chest felt so tight that I was sure I was having a heart attack. All I remember is running as fast as my legs would carry me, not stopping until I had reached the front door of my mother's house.

Of course, once I was in the safety of my home the panic ceased and I began to relax. This horrific experience was diagnosed by my psychiatrist as Agoraphobia, the fear of open spaces. But then these panic attacks began to occur, without warning, three or four times every day, not just outside, but indoors too. Once again my life became a huge misery and I began to dread each day. I could not leave the safety of my home, and dreaded being alone, or in confined spaces. Arrangements were made for me to attend a psychiatric day centre, where my condition could be properly assessed and treated accordingly. I was taken there by taxi every morning at 9:00 a.m. and then home again at 4:30 p.m. I felt so secure there amongst people who were being treated for many different psychological conditions, ranging from drug and alcohol addiction, to anxiety neuroses and other personality disorders. It was good not to feel different and to be amongst people who understood what I was going through. I had abused so many different drugs my condition was difficult to treat. I would abuse anything I was given to relieve tension, and would even take prescribed night time medication during the day, simply because it made me feel nice and relaxed. All medication was withdrawn and I was left more or less to my own devices.

Once it was believed that I was ready to stand on my own two feet, so to speak, I was discharged from the clinic and left to face the cold reality of the frightening world I was living in. One of the most frightening things for me was the fact that the district in which I had been born and had known most of my life, had in fact changed dramatically during the time I had been living and travelling through Europe. Buildings that I had known since I was a child had in fact disappeared completely and had been replaced with newer structures. Neighbours I had known all my life had either died or been relocated to different areas of Liverpool. I was terrified and dreaded the future. I really did think that my use of drugs had caused me to completely lose my mind. I dreaded the future and what the future would bring to me. When I now look back on my horrific ordeal, which I have to say was in-part self-created, I can see that the way in which I was brought up as a child caused many of my hang-ups and made me into the person I had become, psychologically speaking. During this time my father, who was the anchor of the family, had died after a short illness with pancreatic cancer, and now I lived alone with my mother and aunt. I was stuck in a time block with no hope of achieving anything constructive. My music career had gone and there was very little left for me to do. My friends had all abandoned me, and people I had known most of my life did everything they could to avoid me on the street. After careful consideration I decided to end my own life. I was about as low as anybody could be. My only problem was to decide how I was going to do it. As I didn't like any sort of pain or discomfort, I thought the easiest way was to take a fist full of tranquillizers, washed down with a bottle of wine. Needless to say, it didn't work. I'd built up such a high tolerance level over the years that I just slept for 24 hours and woke up with a blinding headache, stomach pains and feeling sick. At least the experience made me realize nothing was actually worth killing myself for. No matter how low you get there's always a solution.

I then began to make some radical changes to my life. I'd not eaten meat or drunk milk since I was 11 years old, so my diet was the first thing I had to consider. I'd lived on an extremely frugal diet for some years, and now I had to explore healthy foods and put some nutrients back into my body. I also realized that I had to change the way I'd become accustomed to thinking about life in general. Instead of being influenced by my mother, and constantly being reminded that I should be more like my brother, Alby, I had to start thinking for myself, try harder to be myself, and not worry that I wasn't like him in any way whatsoever. I set about convincing myself that I was ok the way I was. When I reflected on my life, I realized that I had always been made to feel different. At that time my brother was a fairly successful business man. He had two engineering shops, a nice house in a fairly opulent area of Liverpool, UK, and drove expensive cars, BMWs, Jaguars or Daimlers. He was and still is an extremely conventional-type of guy, where as I always had long hair and wore tatty denims etc. I had to convince myself that there was nothing whatsoever wrong with me, apart from numerous hang-ups, an anxiety neurosis and many other complexes that I was certain I had acquired as a child from the way my parents treated me. I had to realize that there was absolutely nothing wrong with me, regardless of what other people thought. I know self-praise is no recommendation as they say, but I wasn't so different to thousands of other guys my age. Nonetheless, I was still the black sheep of the family, and I was determined to change peoples' perception of me.

In the 1960s meditation was made fashionable by the Beatles who became devotees of the Maharishi Mahesh Yogi, the innovator of Transcendental Meditation, or TM as it was popularly known. In the 1960s I had attended a talk given by the Maharishi at a top London hotel. This had been an inspiration to me at the time, but like so many others at the height of the so-called "Flower Power" era, I had used it, primarily because I thought it was "cool". This was another problem; I didn't really know who I was. Over the years I had created so many personality facades that now I didn't feel comfortable with myself. I found it difficult to interact with other people, and as a consequence I now had very few friends. I was determined that this all had to change. So, meditation was something I decided to integrate into my recovery programme. I knew that this would be an effective way of rediscovering myself, to give me confidence and to put some semblance of order back into my life.

By the late 1970s I had successfully created an extremely effective programme that I used religiously every day, it would seem with some success. I began to feel much more positive and was then able to glimpse the future with far more clarity than ever before. I was beginning to see some semblance of order to my life and was ready to initiate any changes that were necessary for me to give me some sort of life.

My addictive nature covered an extremely broad spectrum, from drugs to sex. One thing I was going to omit from this book is the fact that I have had five failed marriages and thousands of relationships. But I am now very happy and grateful to be married to Dolly, my best friend as well as my wife. In 1982 I founded the Thought Workshop, one of the UK's first centres for psychic and spiritual studies and alternative therapies. The centre became extremely successful in a very short time and was visited by students worldwide. The Thought Workshop caught the interest of the BBC and Granada television who both highlighted the work I was doing in two separate features.

I sincerely believe that we are who we are today as a direct result of who we were yesterday. I'm glad to say that I have never been happier than I am today living contentedly with my wife Dolly in Padstow, Cornwall with our two little pussycats, Poppy and Elly. With this in mind, I knew that if I could magically turn back the clock, I would not change one thing in my past. For as the yogi masters say, "Life is the constant accumulation of knowledge, the storing up of the results of experience; we reap what we sow, not as a punishment for what we have done wrong, but because the effect must always follow the cause."

Get a Grip and Stay Sane: Self-Healing with the Nadi Technique is in fact the sequel to my book *The Holistic Way: Self-Healing with the Nadi Technique*, a unique and extremely effective self-healing system, consisting of various holistic techniques to promote harmony and balance in the body, mind, and spirit. *Get a Grip and Stay Sane* consists of life enhancing methods designed to improve your life psychologically, emotionally and most certainly spiritually. Here I have made a detailed analysis of the cultivation of self-awareness, with the sole intention of reprogramming the mind. In the book I have also offered constructive advice on how to deal with hang-ups, phobias and anxiety neuroses, all of which I have had to endure from my early childhood. The book also highlights the hang-ups frequently imposed upon us by our parents, with a detailed exploration of the metaphysical as well as the psychological implications created as a direct consequence of the way in which we are brought up, right down to the colours we are forced to wear, and the food we are encouraged to eat. The Nadi Technique is an eclectic mix of Eastern and Western methods that also consider ancient yogic practices that are as effective today as they were when they were used thousands of years ago. Over the years I have integrated these methods with others I have also created, which thus culminate into a self-healing system that has always worked for me and which I have used in workshops worldwide. It is not necessary to use the entire programme, as I have formatted it to allow you to use the methods that serve your purpose. In fact, I would advise you to choose the treatments with which you feel comfortable and which work well for you, and then to formulate your own self-healing programme. You may even feel a need to create your own treatments to integrate into the Nadi System. Do whatever is necessary to make it work for you.

My wife Dolly has had many years' experience in corporate hospitality, organizing major events throughout the UK, including arranging menus etc., and is also an experienced interior designer with a flair for colour and the way colour influences and affects our lives, psychologically as well as metaphysically. Her input into the Nadi Technique has been invaluable and is now an essential part of the whole Holistic Programme. In fact, Dolly has created food recipes that have helped us both over the years, and which she also uses in the numerous seminars and residential weekend courses we have put on all over the UK. As I have previously said, I stopped eating meat when I was around the age of eleven, and I have not taken milk in any form since I was a very young child. I have always believed that a non-meat diet is essential for the maintenance of the body's harmony and balance and to promote equilibrium in our spiritual life. It is my belief that if we are ever to live in harmony with the planet and all other life forms on it, then we need to develop respect for the animal kingdom as a whole and begin to see that animals are not here to be exploited by us humans, the so-called intelligent species. After all, to use a now clichéd aphorism "You are what you eat!" The majority of meat eaters would in fact stop eating meat if they had to slaughter the creature themselves. It should also be borne in mind that "you can't stroke an animal with one hand and pick its bones with the other" which is exactly what the majority of carnivores do.

The Nadi Technique is a unique holistic self-healing system for energizing the body to encourage optimum health, thus maintaining balance in our body with the sole intention of improving the overall health. It encourages a healthy balanced diet, correct breathing, positive thinking and attitude, and also helps with the elimination of bad habits, addictions, hang-ups and phobias.

The contents of this book are about changing the way you think as well as the way you act. Thoughts crystallize into habits and habits solidify into circumstances. We always want to change our circumstances, but the majority of people are reluctant to change the way they think, and so in accordance with the Great Law of Attraction they are always bound to circumstances.

Working on the premise that the human organism is an electromagnetic unit of incredible power, the Nadi Technique is an extremely effective self-healing system for maintaining balance in the body with the sole intention of promoting a healthier and longer life.

The Nadi Technique sees the body as a carefully laid-out map, permeated by an intricate network of channels. These channels are called "Nadis", and it is along these Nadis that energy constantly flows, maintaining the body's equilibrium, psycho-logically and physically. As a direct consequence of stress, poor diet, incorrect thinking, and many other reasons, the energy moving along the Nadis congests or solidifies, thereby restricting its relentless flow. This blockage impacts upon the corresponding anatomical part of the body causing a break down in the overall health. A visit to an acupuncture practitioner or even reflexologist usually helps to resolve the problem. Although the principles of acupuncture and reflexology are the same, breaking down the blockages, the methods are different. The Nadi Technique works at a completely different level and includes a broad spectrum of treatments. Some of the treatments included in the Nadi Technique address health issues purely at a physical level, whilst others treat health problems caused at a more subtle level. Combined they culminate into an effective healing force that can also be used on your pets, with great success.

Get a Grip and Stay Sane is the perfect handbook with a step by step guide to right thinking, good health and self-realization, and is an integral part of the self-healing process with the Nadi Technique.

Nadi defined

The majority of Holistic enthusiasts are familiar with Meridians, but only a minority will know exactly what a Nadi actually is. The word Nadi simply means "nerve" or "river", at a more subtle level, and it is one of an extremely extensive network of channels that support the Meridians throughout the subtle anatomy. A Meridian is equated with the trunk of the tree, and the Nadis the branches. As explained above, the Nadis work in the relentless transportation of Prana throughout the subtle anatomy, maintaining balance and equilibrium of the overall health. When a blockage occurs in one or more of the meridians, there is some evidence to suggest that the blockage may have first occurred in the corresponding Nadi, and so regular maintenance of the Nadi system, in the same way that an automobile has a regular service to ensure its mechanical reliability, will maintain a consistent flow of Prana throughout the entire system. The Nadi Technique is not only an extremely effective way of treating a health condition once it has occurred, but also working on the premise, prevention is far better than cure, an excellent process for maintaining the overall health of the network of Nadis, thus ensuring that problems do not occur.

Although as the book later explains there are three major Nadis, the entire subtle anatomy is permeated with thousands of minor and major Nadis that appear, to all intents and purposes, like the wire framework upon which a sculptor moulds his clay. The network of Nadis also supports the seven major chakras, the energy vortices, by conveying Prana from the chakras to the organs of the physical body. The whole thing is an extremely intricate process that does need to be regularly maintained in order to keep the physical body, mind and spirit healthy and well balanced. The Nadi Technique streamlines the subtle anatomy and affects the electromagnetic atmosphere around the body, the outward representation of inner balance or imbalance, whichever the case maybe. The network of Nadis can also be influenced by the mental process of meditation that has the profound effect of re-aligning the Nadis and maintaining their compatibility with the Meridians, the major channels. Meditating every day also helps to maintain psychological balance, alleviating stress and anxiety, two of the main causes that impact upon the stability of the individual Nadis, and preventing the free-flowing Prana from reaching the corresponding components of the physical body. And so, the Nadi Technique is primarily about encouraging optimum health by maintaining overall balance in the body.

Billy Roberts
October 2016

Chapter 1

Decluttering

Step 1: Assessing psychological and emotional rubbish

As well as filling our minds with intelligent and very often useful data, along the way we also acquire a lot of useless stuff, stored securely away somewhere in the subconscious areas of our mind. Unlike a computer in which we can choose where data is stored, to be accessed when needed, the neurological compartmentalizing of data is mostly inaccessible until for some reason it spontaneously filters through into the conscious mind. Although we don't realize it, an awful lot of this useless data causes many of the problems we encounter during our lives. It influences the way we feel about ourselves and very often deprives us of self-esteem, and occasionally encourages us to make wrong decisions; causes us to be indecisive, and generally wears us psychologically down. Psychologists, psychotherapists etc. may very well disagree with what I am saying, but I have gleaned this information from my own direct experience and not from psychology text books. We are all born with the potential to be spontaneous, dynamic, charismatic and successful in life; and once this is fully realized then you should understand that the only thing that is stopping you is the clutter you have acquired on the long road from childhood to the present day. It's now time to clear all the rubbish out and begin to re-programme your own mind, thus filling it with the data of your choice; data that will empower you and motivate you towards success and happiness. "That's all very well," I can hear you say, "but that's easier said than done!" There you go again, making negative statements and adding to the already pile of useless data in your subconscious mind. In fact, every negative statement you make suffices to empower the negative side of your mind even more. A simple mantra such as "Every day in every way I am feeling better and better and better," helps to encourage you towards being more positive and dynamic. For example, an individual who is accustomed to being down in the doldrums every Monday morning is someone who has programmed their mind to be so on a regular weekly basis. On the other hand, getting out of bed earlier than usual on a Monday morning, standing at the end of the bed and throwing your arms out in front of you in a jubilantly triumphant manner, announcing out a loud "It's a wonderful, wonderful Monday morning," will in time really make all the difference to the way in which you perceive your Mondays in the future. Of course, it's not as simple as all that, as you will most probably know, because you need to actually feel what you are saying as opposed to just making the statement out loud; otherwise, it becomes just the intoning of a phrase that produces no real effect on the mind. In saying that, as well as helping to promote an almost hypnotic state or consciousness, intoning a meaningful phrase repetitiously produces an effect upon the subconscious mind, as in the case of chanting a specific mantra in meditation. In the same way that someone can affectionately encourage you to do a specific task by helping you to believe that you are very capable of mastering it, the process of talking to yourself can also be a constructive way of encouragement, and is in itself a subtle form of meditation. A hypnotherapist will instil in a patient the idea that he or she wants to implant in the patient's mind, using a sort of psychological placebo method. This process is frequently used by a mother to encourage confidence in her child who has low self-esteem. The child trusts what his or her mother is saying and therefore believes that it is true. This technique of psychological implantation is extremely powerful and works in exactly the same way as when a mother rubs the pain away from her child's knee after it has fallen over. Within seconds recovery is spontaneous, and with the pain magically rubbed away, the child stops crying and runs off to carry on playing with its friends.

Initially, whether you believe in yourself or not is unimportant when performing in front of other people. Creating a well-rehearsed facade to fool people into believing that you are confident is something that a professional poker player is quite proficient at doing. In other words "Bluffing" is a prerequisite for confidence building and helps to encourage real confidence and strength of character. This may all sound quite ridiculous to someone who already possesses an abundance of confidence, and may sound quite frighteningly impossible to someone who is extremely shy and lacking in confidence, but it really works. You can spend lots of money on hypnotherapy, workshops on confidence building and many other methods available now online; but to achieve it yourself is much more rewarding and will last forever.

As a child I lacked confidence, and because my parents never really encouraged me to overcome my insecurities I was always left to my own devices. When I began working as a musician in a rock band sometime at the age of 14, I always made certain that I stood at the back so nobody noticed me. I had lots of hang-ups and insecurities at that time with absolutely no hope of curing them. In fact, because of my lack of confidence I missed out on numerous career opportunities. De-cluttering your mind and re-programming it is not as difficult as it sounds. You may think it sounds far too easy for it to work, but although the technique itself is very simple, the process does require you to believe in it, otherwise you will defeat the whole object of the exercise, which after all is to encourage confidence in you by re-arranging the way you have become accustomed to thinking about yourself.

Step 2: Mirror

Sit in front of a full length mirror and spend a little time making a detailed observation of the way you look.

Try to be as objectively honest about yourself as you can. Be critical over the way you look almost as though someone else is doing the criticizing.

First of all, focus for a few moments on all your features you are not happy with, such as the shape of your nose, your lips, your eyes, and the shape of your ears.

Having spent some time making a detailed analysis of all the things you don't like about your face, now try and see these features as parts of you that cannot be changed. In fact, with some degree of honesty spend some time looking critically at each of your features.

Now, look at yourself with some admiration as a whole person, turning your head slightly to note your profile. Be perfectly honest with yourself, is there anything at all you would really and truly change if you could. If you are absolutely honest with yourself the answer to that should be NO.

Make a note of both the things you like about yourself and all the things you don't like about yourself. You should be pleasantly surprised.

Lack of confidence is purely subjective and very often has nothing whatsoever to do with anything outside of your own mind. You must realize that your insecurity is based on how you think other people perceive you and nothing more. Some days you are bound to feel more insecure than others, and some days you may feel really good about yourself. That's a natural fact of life and even the most confident of people feel bad about themselves some days. If you've grown up with your mother always telling you are beautiful, or handsome, then in your adult life you are really going to think that you are, whether or not it is true. The things our parents instil in us when we are young are the very building blocks of confidence or lack of it, depending that is on what is said to you and how exactly it is said. A person whose parents have drummed into them that they are absolutely beautiful or special will nearly always grow up feeling different, very often to their detriment. However, in some cases what we are told by our parents can produce arrogance and vanity. Success too is nearly always produced in a person by the way they have been treated in his or her childhood. A deprived childhood is very often motivated to do better and develops the *will* to succeed in later life so he or she can provide for their children the things that they never had when they were young.

Step 3: Self-analysis in preparation

For this you will need a writing pad and a pen.

Sit comfortably with pen in hand, and make a note of everything you can think of that as far as you are concerned

5

makes you unhappy, insecure and which contributes to your general lack of confidence. At this point only turn your consideration to your insecurities and not to the way you would like to really be.

Having made a list, no matter how long or short, spend ten minutes or so studying it, adding things or making changes to it. This is not as easy as you think. This process involves a little bit of honesty and seeing yourself objectively. Go over the list several times until it is fixed firmly in your mind. Are the things on the list things that can be easily rectified? For an example, are you shy or self-conscious, particularly in crowds? If this is one of the things on your list try to take a look at every detail of your self-consciousness, and try to understand why you are like this.

Do you possess all sorts of phobias or obsessions to the extent that you always feel miserable and out of it? Have you always had low self-esteem and now find it unbearable? Is your life one long catalogue of ups and downs, with one problem after another?

It is important to look at the list you have made at least once a week. This will allow you to assess your progress as you move through the programme, and to see which of the things on your list still cause you some difficulty. Although it may take some time you will be able to delete each one as it has been dealt with. Helping you to overcome some of your insecurities is very often as simple as learning to breathe properly, an integral part of the Nadi Technique.

Step 4: Breathing correctly

The majority of people take very little notice of their breathing. In fact, breathing is quite natural and is therefore taken for granted. We never stop breathing whether we are asleep or

6

awake. In fact, it is an essential part of our being. The majority of people are indifferent about breathing and never pay any attention to it. But taking a few deep breaths in the morning can set you up for the day more so than a hearty, healthy breakfast. In fact, we can survive without food for weeks and even months, and exist without water for days, but only a couple of minutes without air.

It is this vitally important respiratory process that keeps us alive. Our life begins with that very first breath and ends with the last.

Few people actually realize that many of our hang-ups, physical as well as mental defects are caused by incorrect breathing. Breath is in fact life, and life is solely dependent upon breath.

The condition of every single component of which our body is composed is dependent upon a healthy bloodstream. The air we breathe replenishes the blood making it more efficient in the relentless process of maintaining the health of the nerves, cells, tissues, glands, skin and all the organs that are vital to the health of the body. All the activities of the body from the digestion to the process of thinking are maintained by the oxygen supply to the body, and even the condition of our teeth, hair, bones, eyes and nails is dependent upon the air that we breathe. Breathing correctly encourages a more efficient flow of oxygen through the bloodstream and revitalizes the whole body, clearing the mind and encouraging alertness.

In the western world we are taught from a very early age to breathe by expanding the upper part of the chest, when in actual fact we should be breathing from the diaphragm. It is now believed that incorrect breathing is the root cause for many of childhood health conditions as well as many behavioural problems. In his book *Organizing the Human Body*, morphologist Dr

Philip Rice, stated that 55 percent of delinquency in children is caused by shallow and incorrect breathing and lack of fresh air.

When the blood is deficient in Oxygen an excess of poisonous carbon dioxide occurs as a direct result. A lack of oxygen in the bloodstream produces fatigue and an inability to concentrate. When allowed to become habitual, shallow breathing is one of the causes of innumerable ailments ranging from nervous disorders to colds and throat infections. A poor posture, such as stooping shoulders, produces shallow breathing, poor complexion, impaired vision, lack of confidence and lethargy. Dr Philip Rice also suggests that a person needs to take at least 60 deep breathes a day in order to maintain a healthy body.

As someone who has suffered with Bronchiectasis since I was 3 years old, I know only too well the importance of regular deep breathing. In fact, I have always spent half an hour every day, regardless of where I am or what I am doing, breathing slowly and deeply. Deep measured breathing is also extremely effective in quelling the flow of adrenalin when one is in the grip of a panic attack. It calms the nerves and promotes serenity.

People who spend their days working on a computer very rarely enjoy good health and nearly always have a bad posture. Deep rhythmic breathing is an extremely effective way of energizing the body and restoring its vitality. In his book Be Happier, Be Healthier, Gayelord Hauser suggests that deep rhythmic breathing is also more important for the health than good food. This is the very reason why Yogis eat very little and practise Pranayama, a form of deep rhythmic breathing, used to control the levels of prana coming into the body.

Prana

In the eastern parlance of yoga the word Prana is used to describe all energy in the universe. In his book Science of Breath, Yogi Ramacharaka also explains that Prana is the principle responsible for the integration of the cells into a whole. In other words it binds everything together; and when it withdraws from the body through the natural aging process, the body dies and then disintegrates. It is the Yogi's belief that retaining larger amounts of Prana in our bodies, encourages good health and encourages our longevity, and allowing us to enjoy healthier lives.

Although Prana is in the air that we breathe, it is neither the air itself nor the oxygen in the air. Although it is in all forms of matter, it is not matter itself. It is present in water and in the majority of healthy food substances we eat, but it is neither the water itself nor the food we consume. Prana is essential for the maintenance of life, and without it we die. Prana is not only referred to by Yogis as a vital cosmic energy, but it was also known to many of the ancient esoteric schools of Egypt, Tibet and China. It is mentioned in the book of Genesis as the mysterious energy, Neshemet Ruah Hayim that God breathed into the nostrils of Adam. Here the literal meaning is "Breath" or the Spirit of Life.

Breath control allows you to obtain the absolute best from the air that you breathe, which not only revitalizes all the major organs of the body, but also promotes calmness in the nervous system and serenity of the mind.

Step 5: Breathing

Although there are extremely advanced pranayama exercises, in the initial stages you would be advised to use the simplest methods, and never strain your breathing or make it a labour, as this merely defeats the whole object of the exercise.

Until your breathing capacity increases, you should begin with two basic breathing exercises. One is deep breathing, and the other is measured breathing.

Begin with deep breathing, taking great care not to over-breathe as this may cause you to hyperventilate. This is best carried out in the garden or by an open window.

Standing up, slightly stoop forward with your hands on your thighs. Slowly expel all the air from your lungs, and then slowly inhale a complete breath, straightening your spine as you do, making sure that when the breath inhalation is complete you are standing perfectly straight.

Slowly allow your body to stoop slightly as you exhale all the air from your lungs, when this procedure is complete, inhale once again, slowly straightening your spine, again making certain that when the breath is complete you are standing up straight with your legs slightly apart.

Repeat this approximately five times, more if you feel you can.

For the best results practise this deep breathing exercise upon rising every morning.

The value of deep breathing is immense; better still if you live by the sea. As long as the air is blowing from the sea as opposed from inland, the prana will be prevalent and drawn-in with each breath. In fact, breathing in the sea air, to the extent you can taste the salt at the back of your throat, is an excellent cleanser for the bronchial tubes and the lungs themselves. It also stimulates the brain and the bloodstream, and is an excellent tonic when you are suffering from depression or recovering from illness. In fact, Victorian physicians used to prescribe a holiday by the seaside for patients recovering tuberculosis or other respiratory diseases. They believed that some geographical seaside areas had that certain "something" in the air that would hasten recovery. Even though prana is outside the parameters of scientific thinking, many scientists are now beginning to accept that there is something other than oxygen in the air that we breathe.

Step 6: Rhythmic or measured breathing

Once you have mastered the art of deep breathing, you should then turn your consideration to Rhythmic breathing. There are two ways of practising rhythmic or measured breathing; one is with a little visualization, and the other is not.

Prana responds immediately to visualization, and when carried out properly it serves as a tonic to the whole system.

Sit on a straight back chair with your eyes closed, and spend a few moments focusing your attention on your breathing and the rhythm of your heart.

Now, ascertain your heart beat by placing your middle and your ring fingers on your pulse, and count, 1,2,3,4,5,6: 1,2,3,4,5,6 and so on.

We base the rhythmic time upon each pulse beat corresponding with the beat of your heart. And so for this exercise the inhalations and exhalations should be to the count of six pulse beats, and the retention and between breaths should be to the count of three pulse beats.

Once you have established the rhythm of your heartbeat, with your eyes still closed, place your hands on your lap and then inhale very slowly a complete breath counting six pulse beats, hold it counting three, and then exhale counting six, and so on.

Continue this for as long as is necessary to make the mind quite.

Next, following the same process, with each in-flowing breath imagine streams of intense white light coming through your nostrils and then into your lungs, on the breath retention see the intense white light circulating your solar plexus, and then on the exhalation discharge all the toxins from your body in a cloudy grey mist. Repeat the exercise for as long as is comfortable, and then relax for a few moments.

On the conclusion of the exercise it is always a good idea to drink a glass of mineral water charged with prana in the following way. Pour the water from one glass to another, backwards and forwards for a minute or two until it seems to almost come alive. Make sure the glasses are held at least five inches apart so that the water is poured through the air. Pouring the water in this way ensures that it is infused with prana. Water charged in this way also precipitates the prana previously draw-in with the breath and helps with its distribution around the body.

The above methods of breathing also help in the process de-cluttering the mind. In fact, rhythmic breathing is an extremely effective way of calming an anxious, worried mind, and also helps to streamline the way in which thoughts are processed by eliminating negative thinking. Should you find the count of six a bit of a strain, then use the count of four inhalations and exhalations, retaining the breath for the count of two. But never strain the breathing as this will only defeat the whole object of the exercise.

We live to all intents and purposes in a crazy chaotic age of science and technology, where the pace of life is fast and for many very often out of our control. It is little wonder why many people find themselves out of tune with the universe. Rhythmic breathing encourages your attunement with the universal pulse, and also repels the disturbing influence of the negative vibrations of the environment and other people. The concept of rhythmic breathing is by no means new and has in fact been practised by the yogis for thousands of years as an effective means of attuning the mind and elevating the consciousness. For this very reason it forms the very basis of the Nadi Technique. Rhythmic breathing nourishes and cleanses all the components that make up the body making it resistant to the attack of disease.

Chapter 2

Relaxation and posture

Whenever we are in the grip of panic or anxious about something, we are always told by our friends to relax and calm down. Easier said than done you may well say, but really the internal turbulence produced by the sudden rush of adrenalin very often bears no relation whatsoever to what is going on outside of our own brains. Of course we don't realize this when we are actually panicking, and some people are more sensitive than others to panic and are affected more profoundly by the slightest stressful situation. Oversensitivity to the pressures of modern day living can have a disastrous effect upon the nervous system and can even sensitize the brain to respond to the slightest bodily sensation. Once this occurs the person begins to experience frequent panic attacks and will over-react even to the slamming of a car door or the piercing sound of a car horn.

Although the adrenal glands react naturally when a person is in a threatening situation, when the brain has become sensitized the slightest thing can trigger an irrational fear, sending the sufferer into panic mode. If this should occur while he or she is in the bank, the person subconsciously associates the bank as being the cause of the anxiety attack, so they make every excuse to avoid going into the bank. This irrational fear is usually subconsciously moved from one situation to another, until everywhere a panic occurs becomes just another place to avoid. Aversion therapy is an ideal but not an easy way of facing a fear head on. When the fear has been faced over and over again it loses its power and is no longer a threat. This said, aversion therapy is not at all easy to go through, but one can learn to relax to such an extent that it becomes almost second nature. Deep relaxation strengthens the nervous system and empowers an anxious person making them resistant to stress.

You can usually ascertain the level of stress a person is under by their posture and their gait. A depressed or anxious person tends to slouch, and his or her gait is usually slow and deliberate and very often quite clumsy. An anxious person, who has become quite accustomed to having a panic attack on a regular daily basis, tends to walk without moving his or her arms, almost as though subconsciously they don't want to be noticed. This person also nearly always has some difficulty looking you in the eyes when engaged in conversation. His or her complexion is nearly always pale with eyes that are either dull or wide with dilated pupils and sometimes redness on the eyelids.

A tense and anxious person nearly always finds it difficult to relax. Even at the end of a hard day at work, they have great difficulty turning off and relaxing.

Because the mind of an anxious or depressed person is always tired, they nearly always feel physically exhausted. Whether there is a belief in the presence of prana in the air we breathe or not, mental and physical fatigue can be overcome with some very simple and straightforward bodily movements, combined with a little rhythmic breathing.

Step 7: Motivation, exercise, and breathing

The MEB approach consists of three simple steps: Motivation, Exercise and Breathing.

People suffering from depression and anxiety very often lack motivation and drive. Getting started in the morning requires great effort, and so the MEB approach is an ideal way of "kick starting" the brain into taking control. A depressed or anxious person very often has low blood sugar (hyperglycaemia) in the morning, causing some weakness, lethargy and a little dizziness. This alone can trigger an anxiety attack, or lead the sufferer into believing that he or she is having a heart attack; when in actual fact it is physiological response to the way he or she is feeling at that moment. As mentioned earlier a sweet drink or a dextrose tablet usually helps to remedy this. The temptation to stay in bed is often very great when one is depressed or suffering from anxiety. The reluctance to begin the day prevents them from getting up in the morning. It is important not to lie in bed in the morning, thinking negative thoughts. If you're not tired pull back the bedcovers and sit on the edge of the bed, shoulders thrown back and your hand resting lightly on your lap. Take several deep breaths with your eyes closed, resisting the temptation to dwell upon one particular thing. Discipline yourself: prepare yourself for the day: Move your mind away from all bodily sensations, regardless of how you feel. DO IT!

Feel motivated. Pull yourself to your feet and open the window as wide as you can. Standing as straight as you can, with your shoulders thrown back as before, exhale, emptying your lungs completely; hold your breath for a few seconds before slowly breathing-in. While breathing-in gently tap your chest all over; when the breath is complete, tap the palms of both open hands firmly against the chest, and then exhale, forcing the breath through pursed lips. Repeat this just one more time.

I have already earlier explained that we should aim to take at least 60 deep breaths during the course of the day, obviously not all at the same time. This helps to revitalize and replenish the blood stream, thus energizing the entire body. Take a few of these deep breaths while standing in front of the open window, and then get on with the day.

It is important to understand, once depression has been diagnosed by your physician, with the usual routine tests to eliminate thyroid problems or any other health conditions that cause lethargy and feelings of anxiety and depression, and you know for certain that what you are experiencing is all in the mind, so to speak, then you must make every effort to ignore the way you feel and motivate yourself. Depression makes everything in the world around you look dark, grey and ominous. Tell yourself that this is a purely subjective state and is in many ways not at all real. Try your very best to ignore it. If you fail, don't worry, you can try again the next day. And that's the important thing; you must always try again and never, ever give in. I do appreciate to a person in the grip of depression what I am saying may very well sound inane and absolutely nonsense. But you've got nothing whatsoever to lose, and everything to gain. Besides, one of the very reasons I am writing this book is because I have been there.

Focusing and structure

This too may very well sound absurd; but while you are feeling the way you do each day must be planned and given structure. Try not to leave yourself to your own devices by taking each hour as it comes. This is obviously different if you are in a job of work.

In this case apply yourself totally to your work, mentally driving yourself forward.

Having no structure to your day will make you even more vulnerable and susceptible to panic or even deeper depression. Once you are washed and dressed and ready to face the day, clear a floor space in your home, or even better, depending on how nice the weather is, go into the garden or yard and stand as straight as you can, hands by your sides and shoulders thrown back. Make sure your back is straight with your head held high, rather a like a child standing in line before the teacher.

Without bending your legs or moving your arms from your side, using your toes to propel you, spring up and down on the spot for a minute or so, seeing how much leverage your toes will give you. You will be surprised just how high you can actually jump this way. Try not to exert yourself too much, and in any case do this for no longer than a minute, a little longer if you feel you can. Remember, it's important to keep your body straight with your arms by your sides and your head straight with your eyes fixed in front of you.

This exercise is invigorating and in many ways more beneficial than a short walk through the park. As well as exercising the lungs and heart, it stimulates the flow of energy through the Nadis, and encouraging its circulation. When structuring your day it is a good idea to integrate this exercise into your day. This must be done even when you feel lethargic and down in the doldrums.

People who suffer from panic attacks or bouts of acute depression frequently do so in private. It is important to share the way you feel with your nearest and dearest. If you go to work you must share the way you feel and what you experience with your colleagues. At least this way you won't feel vulnerable and afraid of having an attack in front of other people. It's good to share, particularly your thoughts and feelings.

Remember this: the posture of a confident person is completely different to the one who has no self-esteem. Holding your head high with your shoulders thrown back not only makes your feel better, but also alters your whole demeanour and makes you look confident even if you don't feel it. So, get into the habit of walking with your head held high and your shoulders thrown back. A person's gait is in fact his or her personal statement about who and what they are. It says weather they are confident or have low self-esteem; arrogant and self-assured, depressed or sad. The way you think about yourself and the world around you is reflected in the way you walk as well as the way you talk.

Chapter 3

Nostril breathing

The majority of people take breathing for granted. It's something we do without thinking. In fact, even when we are asleep the process of breathing continues without any input from us. Little wonder then why many people simply do not breathe correctly, and frequently breathe through their mouths as opposed to through their noses. Mouth breathing is the cause of many of the diseases with which we suffer today. Children who persistently breathe through their mouths grow up with impaired vitality and weakened constitutions, and in later adult life frequently suffer with chronic respiratory diseases. Apart from this, mouth-breathing causes persistent cold and catarrhal affections. When not in use the mouth should be kept closed throughout the day to prevent infections. The nostrils possess their own protective filters that prevent dust and other foreign particles from entering the lungs. The respiratory organs are unprotected when we breathe through our mouths, and dust mites and germs may enter the lungs unrestricted, without anything to filter the in-flowing air. Apart from providing this extremely essential filtering process, the nostrils also warm the air en-route to the lungs.

Something that is rarely used becomes weak and loses its efficiency. As a small boy, because of the debilitating lung disease I contracted when I was three, I was a mouth breather. When this was investigated by the hospital consultant it was found that because of my persistent mouth breathing, one of my nostrils had in fact closed up. Surgery was carried out to drill the atrophied nostril, thus to encourage me to breathe through my nose. To prevent the nostril from closing again, for six weeks I had to suffer a long narrow tube that ran from my nostril, up the nasal passage and into my throat. My parents had to take me to the hospital three times a day so that the tube could be washed-out with a saline solution, thereby ensuring its cleanliness. I had to learn how to breathe through my nose, and today it's second-nature. So I understand fully the importance of breathing through the nose as opposed to the mouth. We should no more breathe through our mouths than we would attempt to take food through our noses. The majority of people don't realize that they are breathing through their mouths, except after some strenuous exercise, or perhaps when they wake up in the morning with a parched mouth. It may well be that you think you can't breathe through your nose, complaining that you constantly suffer from catarrh or sinus problems. Try this simple test.

Step 8: Nasal pressure testing

Close the left nostril with the thumb of your left hand. Breathe-in deeply through your right nostril, and before breathing out, place the thumb of your right hand under the right nostril, as close to it without actually touching it. Now breathe out forcibly, ascertaining the pressure of the out-flowing air from the right nostril against your thumb. Now repeat the process with the left nostril. Close the right nostril with the thumb of your right hand; breathe-in deeply, and before breathing out, place your left thumb under the left nostril, as close to it as possible, but making sure not to touch it. Forcibly exhale, ascertaining the pressure of the out-flowing air against you thumb.

You will probably have noticed the pressure of the out-flowing air was stronger and more noticeable from one of the nostrils; but if you could feel no air from one of the nostrils then there is more than likely a blockage of some sort. It may only be a temporary blockage as a result of nasal congestion or the aftermath of a cold, so this needs to be repeated over a few day to make certain.

The treatment

Open a window, or even better stand in the garden. Take several deep breaths with your mouth firmly closed.

Now, close the left nostril with the finger or thumb of your left hand, and then inhale and exhale several times, making certain that your mouth is closed. Repeat the whole process with the right nostril. This treatment should be practised morning and afternoon for at least a week or until the problem is remedied. This is not to be confused with the yogic alternate nostril breathing which I will explain next. This treatment is purely to cleanse the nasal passages and free them of any blockage. The action of inhalations and exhalations also precipitates the in-flowing prana.

The use of a gentle inhalant, such as eucalyptus in hot water sometimes helps. Or, if you can, inhale some salt water from the palm of your hand. Not everyone can do this, but it really does help to clear and cleans the nasal passages.

Step 9: Alternate nostril breathing

Although this is not a book about Hatha Yoga, I have always found the alternate nostril breathing exercise extremely good for clearing the mind as well as the nasal passages. It also promotes alertness and clarity of thought and eases tension headaches.

I won't ask you to assume the lotus position, although if you practise yoga and are inclined to do so, then feel free. Otherwise sit comfortably on a straight back chair.

Place the tip of your right thumb lightly against the right nostril and the ring and little finger lightly against the left nostril, without closing either. The index and middle fingers should be together and resting on the forehead, maintaining a slight pressure, between the brows, throughout the exercise.

Exhale deeply and quietly through both nostrils. Now close the right nostril by pressing the thumb against it, and slowly and quietly inhale deeply through the left nostril.

Now close both nostrils, whilst maintaining a little pressure on the forehead with the index and middle fingers, retaining the breath, if you can, for the count of four.

Release the right nostril, but keeping the left nostril closed, slowly and yet fully exhale through the right nostril to the count of four. As this count begins slightly raise the head.

When you have fully exhaled, without pausing, begin to inhale through the same nostril (the right), again to the count of four. The left nostril remains closed.

Now close both nostrils, whilst retaining the breath, to the count of four.

With the right nostril remaining closed, release the left nostril, and inhale deeply through it to the count of four.

Without pausing, slowly exhale through same nostril (left).

Close both nostrils to the count of four, and then closing the left nostril, breathe-in through the right nostril, again to the count of four.

Without pausing, slowly exhale through the same nostril (right) maintaining the rhythm to the count of four, and so.

Now close both nostrils for the count of four.-

Repeat the whole process several times before relaxing.

To avoid confusion it might be a good idea to read through the exercise a few times until you fully understand exactly how it is to be executed.

A few points

When executing the breathing process, on the inhalations the abdomen and chest should only be slightly expanded, and on the exhalations slightly contracted. The inhalation is completed during the count of four. This count may be increased as you become more proficient with the exercise.

You will already have noticed from the previous pages the importance I place upon correct breathing. This not only encourages the free movement of air into the lungs, but it also precipitates prana through the Nadis, the fine channels conveying the vital force through the subtle anatomy. Breath is life, life is solely dependent upon breath. It is during the process of respiration that prana collects in certain bodily centres, from where it is continually dispended throughout the body, maintain harmony, balance and equilibrium.

Chapter 4

The body: a mind of its own

You don't need a book to tell you how difficult it is to pull yourself together when one problem seems to follow another, very often making you feel as though some invisible force is exacting its power over you, and delighting in your misery. And then someone makes the inane suggestion that you should really have faith or even pull yourself together! Well, if you could you most certainly would, wouldn't you? The mind is the common denominator where our lives are concerned and, depending on what frame it is in when we are faced with a decision, once the decision has been taken, there is no turning back! It's difficult to cultivate a positive attitude when everything in your life has gone wrong. Stress is insidious and has a way of slowly wearing you down. In fact, the effects of stress are holistic and affect every part of your being. When you have low self-esteem everything affects you. A stranger's odd glance, a pointing finger, an unfriendly voice will bring you down more, even though the perpetrators of the things responsible for bringing you down most probably never intended them in the way you thought. More often than not it is all in the mind. They do say you are what you eat. This is very true to a large extent. But it is now an accepted and truer fact still that you are what you think. The way you think exerts an extremely greater power over your life than you realize. I am not talking about thinking fleeting, indefinite thoughts, but thoughts that are one-pointed, focused and persistent. The aphorism *"As a man thinketh in his heart, so is he"*. Is so comprehensive as to reach out to every situation and circumstance of our lives. It makes sense then, that if, as the old saying goes, we can think ourselves into an early grave, then we can surely increase our longevity through the same mental process. An individual who always thinks that no good will ever come out of anything he does, is constantly defeating his own purpose. Negative thoughts always produce negative actions, and negative actions more often than not create corresponding circumstances. A person who has become accustomed to thinking in this way, always takes a grim delight in being right about their own persistent failures. Little does this person realize that his or her failure in life originates in their own mind. In fact, we are all the architects of our own destinies by the way we think, and we are constantly peopling our own private portion of space with the thoughts we release. That portion of space can either be filled with the radiating power of success, happiness and good health, or cluttered with misery, failure and the fear of poor health. The longer you dwell in the gloom of negative thinking, the more difficult it will be to transform that gloom into the radiance of positive thinking. To an extremely negative person half a glass of water will always be half empty, never half full. Positive thoughts possess the same power as negative thoughts and work in the opposite way. The power of the mind is in itself neither negative nor positive—it just IS. When you have spent a lifetime thinking negative thoughts, cultivating the process of positive thinking becomes all the more difficult. Although initially you may not be able to stop negative thoughts from passing occasionally through your mind, you do have the power to prevent them from orally be given form.

26

Voicing your fears and apprehensions not only quickens their resonance with the universe, but it also makes others privy to your weaknesses. Once this has been done, your chances of recovering your confidence and transforming your life, becomes all the more difficult.

It is a known medical fact that stress causes many diseases, some life-threatening. And these range from depression, to heart complaints, anxiety to even cancer. A person lacking in confidence has most probably spent a lifetime being that way; and creating confidence when you are not is virtually impossible.

Step 10: Taking control

Some people actually thrive on stress; the adrenalin produced by stress gives them a buzz and gets them through, whilst it causes others to panic and withdraw.

There are a few simple things that will help in the process of taking control; things that the majority of people would not even think about.

Whenever possible sleep in as dark a room as possible, or cover your eyes.

Always sleep in a well-ventilated room, window open whenever possible.

NEVER sleep with your hands behind your head, or your arms above your shoulders. This produces tension and you will wake up in the morning feeling as though you haven't had a good night's sleep.

Because of the magnetic pull of the planets, you should ideally sleep with your feet towards the south and head towards the north.

Before retiring for the night, take several deep breaths.

To allow the skin to breathe, sleep without any clothes on. If you feel a little cold, it is far better to throw an extra blanket on the bed rather than wear pyjamas or a nightdress.

Remembering that more benefit is derived from the sleep that occurs before midnight, whenever possible have an early night.

Unless you suffer from breathing problems, never sleep on more than one pillow, or on a soft mattress. When sleeping the spine should remain straight.

Before sleeping, relax the body as completely as you possibly can.

Common sense should tell you not to eat a heavy meal before retiring for the night.

Never keep flowers or plants in the bedroom at night, as these can take-up the oxygen.

They do say prevention is far better than cure, but taking these measures to ensure a good night's sleep will most definitely encourage a healthier and more rested body, essential when endeavouring to overcome stress.

These are really common sense things to help in the process of self-improvement. I said earlier that depression or stress is an extremely lonely battle, and although it helps when family offer their support, unless they have actually suffered with either, then they really cannot fully understand the impact it has on one's life. The Nadi technique is a system that considers the individual holistically, so instead of treating a single condition, it encourages the healing process with the person on all levels, emotionally, physically as well as spiritually. One has a direct effect on the other, and by treating the whole person as opposed to one single part, harmony and balance is encouraged. Of course, the Nadi Technique may be used even if you are in perfect health and never get stressed. Should this be the case you really should count your blessings. Nonetheless, as I have previously stated, prevention is far better than cure.

Chapter 5

Please don't eat me—I'm a friend!

I made the conscious decision to stop eating meat somewhere around the age of ten. Although I did this against my mother's wishes, I was quite adamant that I did not want to eat something I delighted in looking at in the field on my many Sunday trips to Wales with my parents. What intrigued me also, was the fact that, on taking one of my friends with us during the summer holidays, not only had he never seen a cow or sheep before, (except in a photo or at the cinema) he also had no idea that these were the same creatures he salivated over as he watched his mother take the Sunday roast from the oven, sizzling. I grew up in Liverpool in the mid to late 1950s when the city was still recovering from the battering it had received during the so-called Blitz of the Second World War, and now looking back I fully understand my friend's ignorance, given that, like the majority of families during that period, his family had no transport, and so his recreation area was confined to the war-torn streets and exploring the many bombed-out houses, of which there were many throughout the streets of Liverpool. So, in that regard as a child I suppose I was quite fortunate; we were the only family in the street with a vehicle, albeit an old van, and although like many people we didn't have a television, we did have the luxury of a telephone, primarily for my father's business. But I digress; unlike today in the twenty-first century, with television and the internet, promoting vegetarianism, recipes for those who prefer a non-meat diet as well as the many different non-meat products available in supermarkets and health food stores, in the 1950s and earlier, there was very little choice, and the majority of working class families, struggling to make ends meet, were lucky if they had a couple of scraps of meat to feed the family, usually in a pan of Scouse, the traditional dish of Liverpool. And so, abstaining from eating meat was a little difficult to say the least, particularly that we have always been brainwashed into thinking that meat is good for you and provides the body with all the nutrients, essential for the maintenance of physical health. I haven't drunk milk either since I was about three years old; although that was primarily for health reasons, today I regard the consumption of milk for a completely different reason, which I will clarify a little later.

The on-going debate of whether or not animals have souls is in itself a little futile. From the biblical story of the fatted calf, to the sacrificial slaughtering of a baby lamb, comes the question: who is willing to do the slaughtering and watch the creature struggle until its blood drains away and its heart stops beating, you? I think not! From a spiritual perspective, those who would be willing to do the slaughtering have something essentially wrong with them, and so whether or not animals have souls is completely irrelevant. The way in which we perceive the soul of any living creature must surely depend upon the depth of our own spirituality; and a profound lack of feeling for animals of any kind results in the failure to make a connection with the true essence of the animal kingdom on any level. As my mentor once said to me "You cannot stroke an animal with one hand, and pick its bones with the other." Enough said I think. What he was trying to say to me was, if a person is willing to do the slaughtering, then he or she has the moral right to eat the animals flesh, cooked of course.

Anyway, we can philosophize all we want about the ethical and spiritual reasons for not eating meat, but the truth is, if you are an animal lover and you enjoy your Sunday roast and your crispy bacon, then you will always find no end of reasons to state your case and salve your conscience for why you eat meat. So, it's all a useless exercise. A carnivore does not see the meat on the plate as a living organism, so why should he or she be mindful of it having a soul? Some years ago now I was walking my Old English sheepdog, Harry, in the park, when an elderly Oriental man stopped to stroke him. After exchanging a few pleasantries, he said smiling "This dog would feed my family in China for a month!" The spiritual status of a country must surely be regarded by the way they treat their animals. Not only does Spain delight with the heinous sport of bull fighting, but for some reason best known to themselves, many Spanish people think it's a sport to throw donkeys from the tops of buildings! What in God's name is that appalling festival all about? Spiritual? I think not!

Medical statistics have shown that a non-meat diet does not suit everyone, and that generally speaking vegetarians are less likely to develop heart disease or certain forms of cancer. Back in the early 1970s, the medical journal, The Lancet, stated that a fairly high percentage of people whose work involved handling raw meat, were more likely to contract certain diseases in later life; bladder cancer being one such disease.

The amount of adrenalin produced by a frightened animal on its way to be slaughtered is still present in its flesh, to some degree, even when it has been well cooked. And so, the implications of meat consumption are fairly obvious and always remind me of the age old precept "You are what you eat." This being the case, why not cut out the "middle man", or, I should say, middle creature, and just eat what it eats. Or at least a variation of it.

Milk

The calf is taken away from its mother to be slaughtered for veal, without giving it any sort of a chance to experience and enjoy life, and the excess milk produced by its mother is bottled for your consumption. The list of reasons why a non-meat diet is preferable to the diet of a carnivore is endless, and yet the western world thrives on the exploitation and commercialization of animals.

As a child a Buddhist paediatrician eloquently explained to my mother that the bodies of our prehistoric forebears needed the appendix to help the digestive system to cope with a non-meat diet. The appendix is actually a part of the large intestine. The cecum is a pouch at the beginning of the large intestine, this transition area allows food to travel from the small intestine to the large intestine. The appendix itself is a small hollow, finger-like pouch that hangs off the cecum. Some doctors now believe that the appendix is actually left over from a previous time in human evolution. It no longer appears to be of any use to the digestive system's function. The western world has always been conditioned into believing that meat is essential in the process of providing the body with the correct proteins etc., and that without it we would become anaemic and fall into poor health. As I have already stated, a non-meat diet does not suit everybody, the Dali Lama being one such example. He apparently has a health condition that necessitates a meat diet.

And so, in my opinion—and it is only my opinion—there is life in everything, to some greater or lesser degree; and where there is life there is essentially a soul. Animals belong to a different life system, and although they do not speak the same language as us, make no mistake about it, they most certainly understand us more than we understand ourselves. They make the effort, why can't we make the effort to afford them the respect they so badly deserve. We need animals far more than they need us!

The Nadi Technique also has a strong consideration for what we eat, and a non-meat diet is much better for the overall health. A non-carnivorous diet raises the vibrations of the soul and encourages the assimilation of prana throughout the Nadis and subtle anatomy. Milk is mucus forming and has a negative effect on those who suffer with respiratory conditions, such as asthma or reoccurring bouts of bronchitis. Although Soya milk does not agree with everybody, it is far better for you than cow's milk. When I was a child my hospital consultant suggested to my mother that I should drink goat's milk, as this proved beneficial to anyone suffering with lung problems. It has fewer mucus forming properties and is therefore less offensive to the body. I simply refused to have milk as a child. I have always been attuned to my own body, and from a very early age I realized that having a chest infection did not always make me feel unwell. Once the Nadi Technique has been integrated into your personal development programme, it will make you more attuned to your own body and the way it functions, thus encouraging a greater awareness of its health and vitality to develop as a direct consequence. The majority of meat eaters wrongly assume that a vegetarian diet is boring, and that vegetarians live solely on vegetables. This is perhaps one of the greatest misconceptions about vegetarians. Not only is a vegetarian diet healthier in every way than that of a carnivore, but it can be extremely delicious. Of course, it would not be advisable to suddenly radically change your diet by not eating meat, when you have spent a lifetime of eating the flesh of animals. It needs to be done slowly, one step at a time. Your diet should also be supplemented with a sustained release B12 capsule. I also recommend a daily dose of Bee Pollen Granules, half a teaspoon to begin with. These can either be taken directly from the spoon, or sprinkled over cereal. Bee Pollen Granules have an acquired taste, and so you would probably prefer them taken with food. The health value of Bee Pollen has been scientifically supported by various researchers over the years. It has a holistic effect on the body and supports the immune system helping to fight off infection. It is anti-carcinogenic; it improves the mobility of arthritic joints; it encourages brain activity and improves the performance of the memory. It also encourages lung function and their overall capacity in asthma and other respiratory sufferers. There has also been evidence of Bee Pollen shrinking the prostate in sufferers of benign prostatic hypertrophy, a condition that can become apparent in men over the age of forty. There is no disputing the holistic value of Bee Pollen that can either be taken in granule form, or if you find the taste offensive, it is available in capsules.

A none-meat diet encourages the assimilation of prana through the Nadis, promoting stability and equilibrium through the subtle anatomy. The long term effects of a none-meat diet on the health always prove to be quite remarkable.

Anyway, the more I see of people, the more I love my two cats, Elly and Poppy.

Chapter 6

The ancient water cure

I have explained elsewhere that water is a conduit for prana, and that water can actually be charged with selected colour vibrations with the sole purpose of treating specific health conditions. Apart from this method of using water, as a way of treating illness, water treatments have been used for thousands of years by yogic masters, even though the concept is comparatively new to the western world. The Pranic content in bottled water is extremely low, and is non-existent in boiled water. I have already explained that by pouring the water through the air, from one glass to another, several times, it is revitalized and becomes "alive" with Prana. Drinking water that has been revitalized in this way, is a powerful tonic to the system and also encourages the movement of Prana through the Nadis.

To Eastern Yogic masters, water is Nature's great restorative force, and its liberal application, internally and externally, is essential for the maintenance of the health and vitality. Even the animal kingdom recognizes the necessity of water for the maintenance of bodily health, and not just for the process of hydration. The therapeutic values of Prana have been known to eastern masters for thousands of years, and although in the western world, Prana as a universal principle, has only previously been known to the practitioners of Yoga, knowledge of it is becoming more and more apparent. Prana is a universal

THE ANCIENT WATER CURE

principle of energy that can be obtained from food, as well as water and air, and then transmuted and converted into other forms of vital energy, to strengthen and invigorate the body and promote health and strength. Although the western world is becoming more educated to the daily intake of water, the majority of people drink very little water throughout the day, and the only fluids they drink are coffee, tea, coca cola, beer or wine, with very little thought to the essential irrigation of their bodies. As the body suffers as a direct consequence of the lack of water, so too does it impact on the Nadis and the subtle anatomy. The Nadi Technique considers the holistic healing energies of water, internally and externally. Although it varies from person to person, on average our bodies are made up of 60 to 70% of water. Water flushes toxins from major organs and transports nutrients to the cells. It provides moist environments for ear, nose and throat tissues, and generally keeps the body in good working order. And so as long as the physiological needs of water are maintained, the health of our bodies will be too. Drinking insufficient amounts of water each day causes dehydration. Even a little dehydration makes us feel lethargic and out of sorts. It is best do drink at least 1.9 Litres of water a day, or 8 glasses throughout the day. Amongst many other things, dehydration causes constipation and congested colons, and clogs up the bowels like debris in sewers. The kidneys are also affected when insufficient water is consumed. Water dissolves the food we eat and converts it into its various elements, so that it may easily be transported to other parts of the body where it nourishes and helps to build up every cell. In fact, the medicinal effects of water are well known. Water acts as a tonic, when taken internally or externally. It helps to reduce the temperature when suffering with a high fever, and also prevents dehydration brought about by a fever. It is a known fact in yogic treatments that when cold water is consumed it will reduce excessive heart action while warm water is believed to increase the heart's action. Water increases the secretion of the kidneys, and helps them to more efficiently dispose of the waste matter passing into them. It also encourages the secretions of other organs, encouraging their efficiency. When administered correctly, and at the correct temperature, water is not only a splendid appetizer, but it is also a powerful natural stimulant and an effective antiseptic. Keeping the body hydrated does not only maintain the efficiency of all the organs of the body, but it also keeps the skin, hair and eyes in healthy condition. It is a medical fact also, that anyone who suffers with lung problems derives a great deal of benefit keeping the body hydrated. The Victorians believed very much in the efficacious effects of water to the extent that they even advocated taking cold baths to cure all manner of health conditions. This seemingly torturous procedure is also recommended by the yogic masters who use water for all kinds of self-treatments. It is an ideal stimulant for the immune system and helps to ward off colds, flu and many other debilitating conditions. Apart from all this, when water is used in a specific ways, it encourages the flow of prana through the Nadis.

Although the Nadi Technique's use of water in the treatment of health is sometimes extremely bizarre to say the least, it is extremely effective, and can also be used on our pets. In fact, our pets respond extremely well to the Nadi Technique's treatments, dismissing all possibilities of the "placebo" effect. I will be exploring Nadi treatments for our pets in the following chapter.

I have already explained how specific colours can be infused with prana in the treatment of disease. Although this is by no means a new concept (as it was known to the ancient Egyptians as explained by Edwin Babbett in his book Principles of Light and Colour) for the purpose of the Nadi technique I have modified the treatments.

Step 11: Infusing the patient with prana

For the purpose of this particular treatment you will need seven fairly generous pieces of muslin or voile, each in a colour of the spectrum.

For obvious reasons, other than applying the treatment to your pet, for the sake of hygiene, it should, I suppose, only be used on family members. And if treating yourself, you will need to enlist the help of your partner.

When you are feeling out of sorts, or perhaps recovering from the flu or some other health condition, your immune system will greatly benefit from an overall boost. The same applies to a dog or cat who nearly always finds this treatment quite pleasant. As I have previously said, for reasons you will soon see, this extremely specialized treatment should only be applied to a family member or pet.

Before beginning the treatment, fill a bowl with water, and using a drinking glass, pour the water from the bowl to the glass, through the air, backwards and forwards for three to four minutes, until the water comes alive. This ensures the precipitation of the prana in the water. When you have done this, place the several pieces of muslin in the water and leave them there for five minutes. Ring-out each piece, thus getting rid of excess water in preparation for the treatment.

Lie the patient on his or her tummy, and place the different coloured (now damp) muslin strategically along the spine. Begin with the red muslin at the coccyx, the orange in the next position, the yellow in the next, and so on, until the seven colours are laid out more or less corresponding with the positing of the major chakras. You may find it necessary to fold the individual pieces of muslin into strips so that they fit across the person's back.

Now, lower yourself into a comfortable position, allowing easy access to the different coloured muslin. Then, inhale a complete breath, and placing your mouth as close to the red muslin as possible, without touching it, blow gently into it, until all the breath has been expelled. Once this has been completed, inhale a complete breath and repeat the whole process again. In fact, apply the blowing treatment three times, ensuring that a complete (deep) breath has been taken.

Repeat the same breathing process with each piece of coloured muslin, beginning with the base of the spine, and then gradually working your way along the spine to the head. The muslin corresponding with the throat chakra should be placed on the back of the neck, and the muslin corresponding with the brow chakra should be placed on the back of the head. The muslin corresponding with the crown chakra should be placed on the crown of the head.

Once the entire treatment has been completed, the hands should be moved along the spine, from the head to the coccyx, with a slow sweeping motion, and without actually touching the person's body. Repeat the sweeping treatment several times.

As with all treatments, the patient should hydrate his or her body by consuming a full glass of water charged with prana. Apart from helping to revitalize the body, this also has a cleansing effect upon the system, as well encouraging the efficiency of the healing force.

Although somewhat different to other complementary treatments, it is one that is extremely effective in soothing painful and inflammatory conditions, and also helps to promote serenity and calmness.

Step 12: Treating fatigue

Assuming that there is no underlying physical cause for the fatigue, and that you have undergone all the tests necessary and your medical practitioner has eliminated any serious health problems, the following treatments will help greatly, by encouraging the movement of prana through the Nadis in the lower extremities. I personally find the first treatment extremely uncomfortable, but with a little perseverance, after the first couple of minutes results will be achieved.

For this treatment you will require two bowls large enough to accommodate your feet. Fill one bowl with warm water, and the other bowl with ice-cold water. The warm water should be the hottest temperature you can stand, without burning your skin.

Sit with one foot in the warm water and the other foot in the ice-cold water. Remain like this for five minutes and then change round.

Each foot should be submerged in the hot and cold five times before the treatment is concluded.

This is not the most comfortable procedure and so it may take you a little while to actually get used to it. Once you have you will feel the stimulating benefits in a very short time.

As with all treatments, a glass of charged water should be consumed on its conclusion.

Chapter 7

Healing and the aura

You are a multidimensional cosmic being living in a multi-dimensional universe, in which there are worlds within worlds, each rising in a gradually ascending vibratory scale, from the highest spheres of the physical world, to the lowest dimensions of the great Astral world. Although it is the general consensus of opinion that the physical body is the most apparent of all our bodies, and therefore the only vehicle of conveyance available to us whilst we live on this dense, three-dimensional planet; the human form is radiant, and transcends far beyond the parameters of the visible spectrum. To qualify this, I use the analogy here of pouring hot molten wax into a bowl of cold water. On contact with the cold water the wax molecules slowly begin to solidify, layer upon layer, allowing it to compete with the alien circumstances in which it finds itself. In the same way, on the soul's descent through the manifested worlds of the cosmos, it becomes encased within numerous sheaths, allowing it to exist on the different planes to which it relates, and through which it continues to descend until finally becoming encased within a physical body.

The human organism itself is an electromagnetic unit of incredible power, assimilating, appropriating, modifying and discharging energy, and is thus contained within its own spectrum of colour and light. Chemical energy is converted by the cells of the body into light energy, culminating into what is known in metaphysical parlance as human bioluminescence, and optical phenomenon that is apparent around some deep-sea aquatic creatures—the glow seen around the body that the majority know as the Aura. This metaphysical aspect of our being extends beyond the parameters of the visible spectrum, and is a database of our personal information. You might say that the aura is a blueprint of our life, all that we have done and all that we are going to do. Although aspects of the aura are transitory and therefore change with every passing thought and feeling, there is a predominant part of it that is a blueprint of our true character and this only changes when we embark upon a strict regime of personal development. One could also describe the aura as a bridge of consciousness, connecting our existence in the physical world, to the great supersensual universe. This concept is perhaps easier to comprehend with the analogy of radio and television waves, both of which are transmitted from their respective stations. The clarity of the reception of both is solely dependent upon atmospherics, the strength of the signal, and also the condition and efficiency of the mediums of both apparatus receiving the signals. In very much the same way is our health dependent upon the condition of our aura, whose job it is to help in the maintenance and streamlining of the in-flowing energy. Disease is very often seen in the aura some considerable time before it actually becomes apparent in the physical body, and with an occasional overhaul, the performance and condition of the aura maybe maintained, thus affecting the health of body, mind and spirit. Although the aura is multidimensional, radiating some distance outside of the physical body, we must not forget that it is produced to some degree by the cells of which the physical body is composed, so it therefore internally reflects the external future of the body. We are only now beginning to understand the long-term effects some foods have on our bodies, and with such a wide range of healthy foods available today, more and more people are becoming health conscious in an effort to improve the quality of their lives. By developing a sensitivity to the vibratory tones of your personal energy field, will you then be able to pre-empt any changes that may occur in the future health of your body. The advantages of this really do cover a broad spectrum, and will also help in your overall spiritual as well as physical development.

Step 13: Auric resonance treatment

Sit quietly with your eyes closed and perceive your body as an extremely powerful electromagnetic unit, with outpourings as well as in-flowing energy. As visualization is an integral part of this exercise, it is important to maintain the imagery and not to allow your mind to wander from it even for a moment. Spend at least ten minutes on this part of the exercise, or at least until the imagery is fully established in your mind.

When you feel satisfied that you have consistently maintained this imagery, slowly turn your focus to your breathing; and with the inhalation push your diaphragm out, and on the exhalation pull it in. The rhythm of the inhalations and exhalations is paramount, as this increases the in-flowing prana into the body, stimulating and revitalizing all the cells, tissues, nerves, fibres and muscles that contribute to the maintenance of your health.

Now, try to see your body as though you were sitting in front of it, carefully scrutinizing it; and when you breathe-in see it suddenly light-up as it comes *alive* with energy, and when you breathe-out see it discharging all the toxins that have accumulated over the years, clogging-up the Nadis and restricting the movement of prana throughout your body.

For the next part of the procedure you should sit quietly with your eyes closed, making a detailed mental analysis of your aura. The first part of the exercise should have made any impurities apparent. Look for parts of your aura that appear dull and lifeless, or even devoid of colour. Concentrate on those areas for a few moments before breathing vitality into them, as you previously did. Breathe in deeply, watching streams of vitality infusing the parts you are treating, and as you breathe out, see all the toxins (impurities) being discharged. Repeat this process several times, or at least until you feel the treatment has been successful. Then relax for a few moments longer with your eyes closed.

Remember, as the aura is composed of subtle particles of electromagnetic energy, it responds more effectively to the way you think. Bringing your aura under the conscious control of your mind, has a holistic effect on the whole subtle anatomy, and as a direct result, encourages the self-healing process. The above exercise should be practised at least once a day, preferably before meals. As always, a glass of charged water should be consumed on its conclusion.

Although we are dealing with subtle energies using a purely mental process, it still expends a lot of personal energy; so it is vitally important that you do not exert yourself in anyway whatsoever on the conclusion of the self-treatment procedure.

Step 14: Healing auric fragmentations and leakages
The aura can become fragmented and damaged in various places and for many different reasons, ranging from stress and

worry, to environmental and circumstances. Apart from its many other functions, the aura also serves as an extremely effective protective body, and protects us from invasive environmental atmospheres, as well as from the undesirable thoughts directed at us by other people. As explained earlier, the aura is also an effective data base, containing all our spiritual, emotional, psychological as well as our physical information. This being the case then, once it breaks or becomes fragmented in any way whatsoever, we are automatically left open to the subtle elements. The thought and emotional debris discharged by other people, floats around in the psychic atmosphere, rather like particles of dust in the air. A healthy aura usually repels these subtle particles with great efficiency, and so the majority of people are not in any way bothered by them. However, a damaged aura is quite vulnerable and is unable to repel such intrusions. These debris infiltrate the breaks in the aura and eventually filter their way through into the innumerable channels (Nadis) thus entering the energy system. Once this has been achieved, the psychological and physical health eventually suffers as a consequence. Although not a physical body, the aura interpenetrates the many components that make up the physical body, and so by regularly overhauling the aura, is the health of the physical body maintained. The aura not only responds to mental interaction, but because it is an extension of physical energy, it also benefits from a salt water bath. The salt water has a cleansing effect upon the skin, affecting the aura's innumerable subtle layers, as well as the obvious cleansing effect on the body.

Lie in the salt water bath for at least half an hour, making sure your whole body is submerged right up to your chin. The temperature of the water should be at a comfortable level. Do not contaminate the water with shower gel or any other bathing products. Just relax in the salt water and enjoy its cleansing effect on your entire body.

Do not use anything but the palm of your bare hand to rub the salt water all over your body, massaging it gently into your skin.

On the conclusion of the salt water treatment, take a shower, cleansing your body and ensuring all particles of salt are removed from your skin.

The invigorating effect on your entire body also encourages the subtle energies of the aura to become more streamlined. Although the effects of the treatment are transitory, bathing in salt water at least three times a week, combined with the visualization method previously given, assists in the whole process of stabilizing the aura.

Always bear in mind that the mind itself is the common denominator when dealing with subtle energies. The aura responds very well to the way we think; and with some positive mental interaction, the aura can be cultivated, in the same way that a sculptor moulds his clay. Once the repairing process has been fully grasped, results are achieved almost immediately.

Step 15: Applying auric healing to others

Auric healing is extremely effective in the process of restoring another person's vitality. Administered every day for a week it can produce some startling effects, particularly when a person is out of sorts, or perhaps is recovering from illness. We've all experienced this at some time in our lives; feeling lethargic with a complete lack of energy. Whenever I feel like this I usually find some rhythmic breathing restores my vitality very quickly. This encourages the movement of prana through the Nadis, thus precipitating the healing process.

The person you are treating should lie face-down in a horizontal position, with his or her arms resting comfortably above their head. Before beginning the treatment it is of paramount importance that they are comfortable and totally relaxed. At this point it is a good idea to talk them through some relaxation; instructing them how to relax each part of the body in turn. Once they are full relaxed, begin the treatment. The initial part of the healing process involves the rotating hands treatment mentioned in my previous book, the Holistic Way. This encourages the vibratory movement of each individual chakra; in itself producing an invigorating effect on the entire body.

Begin by placing the left or right hand (whichever comes easier) at the base of the person's skull, on the neck, without touching, and the other hand over that hand, again without touching it.

Slowly rotate the hand closest to the person's body in a clockwise manner, and rotate the other hand in an anti-clockwise manner. In fact, depending on how good your coordination is, you may have to practise this for a while before commencing the treatment.

Spend a few seconds in that position before slowly moving down to the area around the heart. Spend a further few seconds there before slowly moving to the waste line. In fact, it is better, and probably more effective, to allow yourself to be intuitively guided as to the length of time you remain in each position. The same should apply when considering the locations of the chakras you are treating. Instead of concerning yourself with the exact locations, allow your intuition to guide you.

48

Once you have concluded the whole treatment, and have applied it sequentially to each chakra, again without actually touching the person's body, quickly apply the rotational process from head to toe, backwards and forwards two or three times, whichever you feel is appropriate. This helps to seal the Nadis, maintaining the movement of prana for the following treatment. As always, on the conclusion of the treatment a glass of charged water should be drunk.

Step 16: Repairing and sealing the aura

Some people applying this treatment for the first time nearly always dismiss it because of its simplicity. In fact, there is absolutely nothing at all complicated with any auric treatment; and although the Nadi Technique does not require faith, there does need to be a certain belief that it is going to work, especially on the part of the practitioner. And for this treatment you will require several drinking tumblers each in a colour of the spectrum. Although transparent discs will suffice, these are not as effective as the tumblers. Their depth actually plays an integral part in the process of energy transference, and encourages the vibratory motion of the individual chakras. This process has an extremely powerful effect on the aura as a whole and encourages the precipitation of prana throughout the subtle anatomy.

The person you are treating should remain in a horizontal position lying face down; only this time with his or her arms by their sides.

Make sure that he or she is perfectly relaxed by talking them through the relaxation process, from the head right down to their toes. Once they are relaxed and you have their full attention, move to the next part of the treatment.

You should now breathe rhythmically for a few moments with your eyes closed, aware of the in-flowing and out-flowing breath. Mentally see the in-flowing breath as intense white light, and the out-flowing breath as grey fumes carrying all the toxins from the body.

Take the red tumbler and place it base down at the lowest part of the person's spine, as near to the coccyx as possible.

Turn the glass several times in a clockwise manner, and then place your left hand over the top of the tumbler, holding it there for a few seconds.

Still with your hand on the tumbler, inhale a complete breath, and visualize the in-flowing breath now as pulsating red energy. Hold your breath for a few moments, and then mentally breathe the red energy out through the hand you are holding over the tumbler, mentally seeing it spiralling through the tumbler before finally entering the person's body at that location. In fact, repeat this three times.

Now take the orange tumbler and place this in the same way more or less at the sacral centre. It doesn't really have to be in the exact location of this chakra, as long as the same process is applied. Turn the tumbler several times in a clockwise manner. Place your left hand over the top of the tumbler, and allow it to remain there for a few seconds. Inhale a complete breath, this time mentally seeing the in-flowing breath as vibrant orange energy. Now mentally breathe the same orange energy out through the hand on the tumbler, and mentally see it spiralling through the tumbler before entering the person's body at that location. Repeat this three times.

Follow the same procedure with the yellow tumbler, mentally breathing-in the yellow energy, and then breathing it out into the tumbler. Once again, repeat this three times, more if you feel a need.

Follow the same procedure with the green tumbler, the blue tumbler, indigo tumbler, and then before using the violet tumbler to treat the crown chakra, take a few minutes break.

Before positioning the violet or purple tumbler at the top of the person's head, place your left hand on the back of his or her head, and your right hand on the base of the spine. Allow them to remain in their respective positions, before slowly drawing them slowly together along the spine, allowing them to meet in the middle of the back.

At this point, placing the right hand over the left (without touching) proceed to apply the previously shown rotational treatment. Slowly rotating the left hand with a clockwise motion, and the right hand with an anti-clockwise motion, move first to the back of the person's head, remain there for a few seconds, before moving down to the coccyx (base of the spine). Remain there for a few seconds before concluding the rotational process.

Now, placing the violet tumbler on the crown of the person's, apply the same treatment as you have done previously, breathing out as close as you can into the purple/violet tumbler. Because of the position of this tumbler, breathing directly into may be a little awkward. So don't worry too much. As long as you mentally and almost ritualistically apply the treatment to the best of your ability, it will still be effective.

As with previous treatment, on its conclusion the patient should drink a glass of freshly charged water. As I have already explained, water is charged by pouring it through the air from one glass to another, for fifty seconds or more, or until the water sparkles and looks almost alive.

Chapter 8

Mind over matter

The overall health of our bodies is fundamentally dependent on both the food we eat and the way we think. I have said elsewhere that if, as the old saying goes, we can think ourselves into an early grave, then the same must apply to thinking ourselves into a long and healthy life. Although when we are faced with an overwhelming problematic situation, we can't really help worrying about it, simply because you know as well as I, that such problems preoccupy everything we do, making us feel anxious and overall quite miserable. If allowed to persist, such negative thinking eventually impacts on our health. Although now somewhat of a cliché, "we are the architects of our own destinies simply by the way we think." Getting rid of negative habitual thinking is not as difficult as one might imagine. "Easy said than done!" You may well say, dismissively. "When you are in the grip of worry and panic, how can one possibly think positively?" The Nadi Technique has a more subtle approach to this distressing problem, and uses the "imagination" as a key to a relief system, that in time brings about a complete transformation in the sufferer's whole outlook and attitude towards his or her life. This treatment may take longer to work with some people than with others, but results are guaranteed if persistently applied each day.

Let's take a look at what is involved in the process of imagination and how this plays a part in this particular treatment.

52

MIND OVER MATTER

You may well say that you don't have a very active imagination, and that even the simplest of tasks involving your imagination is carried out with great difficulty. Even if this is the case, everybody daydreams at some time during the day. This is one of the mind's release mechanisms and the brain's way of releasing tensions. Staring into space is something we all do at some point during the day. Sometimes our daydreaming is empty and produced by tiredness, and other times it is a way of processing our thoughts and future plans. However, the neurological image-making faculty is quite a powerful organ and not only supports our daydreaming, but also inspires us and encourages us to make plans for our future. Processing the images of the way we would like our life to be is a natural neurological procedure and an ideal way of motivating us. I have said elsewhere that if we can think ourselves into an early grave, then the same principles must apply to thinking our way into a happier, healthier life. Getting a grip of yourself is not as easy as it sounds, especially when you've most probably spent a lifetime thinking in a negative way and always looking on the gloomy side of things. You probably think that using your imagination to bring about such a transformation to your life is just not going to work. However, until you have tried it you really won't know. Besides, using your imagination really does not take much of your time, it's recreational and can be fun. Let's take a look at the process and what is involved.

Relax in a comfortable chair eliminating all possible distractions, such as disconnecting the phone, and making sure you are alone in the house.

Close your eyes and imagine you are alone in your personal cinema waiting for the movie to begin.

While you are waiting for it to begin, focus your attention on your breathing, ensuring that the inhalations and exhalations are evenly spaced. Breathe in and out, allowing your tummy to rise as you breathe in, and allow it to fall as you breathe out.

Now that you are nice and relaxed, imagine the curtains parting and the cinema screen lighting up.

The movie is called *Your Future* and features all the things and people you feel will brighten your future life and make you happy. If this involves money, then see yourself sitting there surrounded by bags and bags of paper money. Watch as you empty all the bags on to the floor.

Now, allow the people who matter to you to enter the room in the movie. See them all laughing with you.

If it's a healthier life you are seeking, see yourself in the movie absolutely glowing with good health. Watch yourself dancing around the room, jumping from one leg to another. Focus on this for as long as you can.

Remember to picture whatever it is you need to make your life better, and focus on this. It is paramount that you project yourself into the movie and feel as though you already have the things you need to make your life happier and healthier.

Make this visualization process an integral part of your day. Set aside at least an hour of your time just to relax and watch the movie of your future life. Remember, you are the architect of your life by the way you think. Should you allow yourself to believe that your life will always be like this and will never get any better, then that's the way it will be.

You must break-free from your usual habit of thinking in a negative way, and begin to think positively. Remember, nothing is permanent, all things eventually pass. It's far easier to think negative thoughts than it is to think positive thoughts. This a known fact. When you are miserable and worried about whatever is going on in your life, it's almost impossible to feel happy without a care in the world. But if you use the process given above on a daily basis, it gradually encourages you to have a completely different attitude to everything. A successful business person does not become successful just by luck or business acumen alone. He or she knows that they are going to succeed and they do not allow anything to deter them in any way whatsoever. They show determination and self-belief in everything they undertake, and it is this that eventually causes them to achieve the heights of success. They are also persistent in their aspirations and endeavours, and they maintain their success by respecting others. They "know" that they are going to succeed. They feel it and taste it as though they already have success and wealth. This is what you need to do. Do not just wish for it. Do not rely on prayer alone. Imagine you are already successful, wealthy and healthy. Begin by seeing yourself in the movie of your future, radiant, healthy, wealthy and happy; and once you have mastered this technique of visualization, bring yourself from the movie, with all the things that have made you healthy, wealthy and successful and in control of your life, and instil it in your mind that you are already like this.

The same visualization process may be used to help you overcome the things that make you anxious and afraid. Using your imagination, create a movie of all the things that cause you to panic and make you anxious. See yourself in the movie in those situations that cause you to panic. This way you know you are in control and nothing can harm you, because you can leave the movie any time you like. However, if you see yourself facing your fears head on, allowing the panic and anxiety to reach its most frightening crescendo without causing you to flee, you are then more than half way to eliminating panic and anxiety completely from your life forever. You must welcome panic. Meet it head on and master it as opposed to allowing it to master you. The same visualization process may be used to rid your body of illness. In your movie, perceive illness and disease in the same way that you perceived the things that made you anxious and afraid. See whatever it is you are suffering with as horrid-looking creatures much smaller and weaker than yourself. See yourself in the movie pounding them into the ground until they become no more than particles of dust blown away by the wind. You must visualize consistently at least once a day for as long as is necessary. Remember, it may take a little time before you see positive results. You need to be persistent and above all else, believe that it is going to work. Visualization is the key to unlocking the immense inherent powers of your mind.

Chapter 9

Addressing irrational fears

When I first came off drugs all those years ago, it didn't take me very long to realize that I had an extremely addictive nature, and was subconsciously prepared to exchange one addiction for another. Once I was free, so to speak, I had to accept the fact that I had been battered emotionally and psychologically. I was insecure, and extremely anxious. In fact, looking back I can now see that I was frightened of facing the reality of a life without the false support of drugs. I had cut myself off from even the people I had known since I was very young, and became reclusive and would not even answer the front door when somebody called. I had no idea who I really was anymore and had to face the cold reality of a future with any artificial support. I had then gone to live at my mother's home, a small terrace house in a superb of Liverpool in the UK, where she lived with my aunt Sadie. Although my mother and aunt cared for me, the very thought of spending my whole life in their care depressed me even more. I wanted desperately to get my life back together. At that point I did not have any clue exactly how I was going to do this, but I knew that it had to be done. I became so obsessed with the idea that I would be like this for the rest of my life, that I found myself having acute panic attacks for seemingly no reason at all. I was having panic attacks two or three times a day and at the same time. It was so bad I found myself watching the clock and waiting for the dread moment to dawn. When I eventually decided to go for a walk and ventured some distance away from my home, I was suddenly stricken by panic. My heart began pounding against my ribs and a tight band around my chest caused me to gasp for breath. My legs were like jelly and I perspired profusely. I thought I was dying and could feel my whole body violently shaking. I took off in the direction of my home and didn't stop until I was in the house and the door was closed behind me. Only then did I begin to settle down; but it took some time for my body to stop shaking and my heart to regain a normal rhythm. This experience was horrendous and I was worried that my years of drug abuse had caused some neurological damage. I was afraid to leave the safety of my home and so resigned myself to remaining indoors. I had already been in various clinics and hospitals for treatment, and now I checked into rehab to enable my psychological condition to be assessed. In other words, I was a veritable mental wreck and as far as I could see, there was no future.

It wasn't until I saw my name on the "Agoraphobia" group list that I realized what was wrong with me. The psychiatrist said that my years of drug abuse had caused a great deal of mental and emotional trauma, and his prognosis was that it would take a long time for my nervous system to heal.

I checked out of the clinic in Liverpool and took a taxi to my home some four miles away. It was then that I decided something needed to be done about my irrational fears. As I have already mentioned earlier in the book, I had studied and practised various forms of meditation in the sixties and decided I needed to create a self-help programme with mediation and relaxation techniques integrated into it.

People who suffer with debilitating panic attacks generally do so almost habitually. Panic becomes an integral part of his or her biological make-up, and they find themselves in what some psychologists refer to as the "adrenalin-fear-cycle", and breaking free from it is horrendously difficult. An anxiety neurosis produces morbid thoughts and feelings as well as all the other physiological sensations. The irrational fears produced by an anxiety neurosis really do make life miserable for the sufferer, and seeing a way out of it is absolutely impossible. Family or friends telling you to "pull yourself out of it", merely worsens your misery. The sufferer knows only too well that if he or she could pull themselves out of it they would.

Situational panic

When a panic attack occurs, shall we say in the bank whilst you are depositing money, (as earlier explained) the bank is perceived as the cause and so it is avoided at all costs. Of course the bank has nothing whatsoever to do with the panic attack which can occur anywhere and at any time, for no particular reason. If he or she can help it, they make every effort to avoid going out altogether, minimizing the possibility of having a panic attack, or so they think. Once you have suffered a severe panic attack, your whole body becomes sensitive to feeling. The sudden sound of a car horn can send a rush of adrenalin surging through your body, causing the heart to pound inside your chest, accompanied by many other physiological symptoms. The majority of people who suffer from panic attacks are always so tense, subconsciously waiting for the next attack. When panic strikes all the muscles in the body suddenly tense even more, thereby precipitating the release of even more adrenalin. If you do suffer from acute panic attacks on a fairly regular basis, then the first thing to release is that the body can only produce a certain amount of adrenalin at any one given time. Most sufferers add panic to panic, thus perpetuating to overall agony of it. The adrenalin-fear-cycle has to be interrupted, and this is done by sending the whole body into complete relax mode as soon as panic strikes. This is probably easier said than done, but not impossible. As with anything worthwhile, practice does make perfect; and the more you practise relaxing the body, the easier it will become when panic strikes.

Welcoming panic

Panic attacks tend to be more intense when you are alone, with the fear of having a heart attack and nobody there to call for medical assistance making it a greater threat. Although not an easy thing to do, you must practise at welcoming a panic attack so that you can learn how to cope with it. I used to have a huge panic attack around 9am, and I became accustomed to it occurring at that time. I would sit tensely, watching the clock and waiting for it to occur. Little did I then know that I was actually making it happen by tensing every muscle, tissue and nerve in my body. Let's take a look at the process of relaxation.

Step 17: Tense and relax

First of all, stand up straight, making the spine as erect as you possibly can, with your arms hanging loosely by your side. Without falling over, allow your body to gradually go as limp and as relaxed as you possibly can, slowly allowing your chin to fall to your chest and your legs to bend at the knees.

60

Relaxing your body even further, slowly fall to your knees, and presenting no resistance, slump slowly to the floor, and remain in that position, totally relaxed with you head turned to one side, feeling as though all the energy has been drawn from your body and you are completely paralysed and totally unable to move.

Remain in that position for at least five minutes, resisting all temptation to move or to respond to any bodily sensations, such as tingling of the skin.

On the conclusion of the five minutes in this position, beginning with your feet and legs, very slowly tense all the muscles in your lower extremities, making your legs more and more rigid as you make your way up to your thighs and then your buttocks. Now, make the muscles in your back and stomach as rigid as you possibly can, slowly allowing the tension to move to your arms, your neck and all the muscles in your face.

Make your entire body as rigid and as tense as you possibly can, maintaining the rigidity for as long as you can bear it.

When you can no longer continue tensing your body, just quickly let go of all the tension and relax all the muscles, nerves, tissues and cells of your body, feeling everything tingle as your body relaxes more and more. Just let go as completely as you possibly can. Remain in that relaxed position for a further five minutes.

Although somewhat exaggerated, this allows you to see just what tension does to your body when allowed to build up during the course of the day. Try to practise this exercise every day, and in no time at all you will be able to relax without even thinking about it. If you prefer, you can go through the same process lying on the floor or even on your bed. Remember, practise your relaxation even when you feel well and not anxious. This brings

61

it more under your control when you're in the actual grip of panic.

Make a list of all the things that frighten you

Sit down and make a note of everything that causes you to panic. This will probably take longer than you think, and as long as you are honest with yourself, you will be surprised as to just how many things really do cause you to panic. Aversion therapy is used by many psychotherapists; and although it can be extremely effective, it is a difficult way to treat your problems. And they are problems, albeit horrendous problems. Aversion Therapy is the process of facing the things that cause you to panic; facing each one and seeing it through until it is no longer a threat. But as long as you instil into your head that all the things that cause you to panic are not permanent, and that they are not an integral part of you, then you will accept that you can and will eradicate all your fears and anxieties that are making your life miserable. Learning to face your fears and the things that cause you to panic is an extremely effective way of overcoming them. This de-sensitizes your nervous system and makes you much more in control of your life. By allowing yourself to be angry with your panic attacks are you able to over-ride them. Instead of giving in and becoming subservient to your panic attacks, let go and be angry with them. This uses up the increased adrenalin that actually causes and perpetuates the panic, making you the controller, so to speak, instead of the one being controlled.

Chapter 10

Treating pain with pain

This may seem somewhat paradoxical, but in the same way that homoeopathy treats like with like, the Nadi Technique treats pain with pain. I have explained that the body is a veritable network of channels called Nadis. The Meridians in acupuncture are synonymous with the trunk of the tree, and the Nadis the branches of the tree. Although the Meridians play an extremely important part conveying energy (Prana) throughout the body, so too do the Nadis help in the relentless conveyance of Prana by supporting the Meridians in the process of the overall maintenance of the health. When a person is suffering with painful inflammation of the joints, as in the case of arthritis, by applying a little pressure at strategic points, where the Nadis converge, until discomfort is felt, the inflammation is relieved. When the pressure is applied several times, over a period of three to four days, permanent relief is very often achieved. Before I continue, I do have to say that a medical practitioner must always be consulted before applying the Nadi Technique. And never stop taking prescribed medication without first consulting your doctor.

Step 18: Ascertaining Nadi location

Lie the patient in a horizontal position, or if easy access can be gained to the affected area, seat them in a comfortable chair.

Gently tap around the painful joint with your middle finger, ascertaining exactly where the Nadi is in relation to the painful inflammation. This is done with the help of the person you are treating who will tell you when he or she feels a little tender.

Once the location of the Nadi has been determined, first of all, apply the palm of one of your hands to that area, gradually increasing the pressure until the person the person tells you he or she feels some discomfort.

Once discomfort is felt, place the thumbs of both hands on the same area, apply a little pressure, before slowly rotating both thumbs in a clockwise manner, gradually increasing the pressure. As in the previous part of the treatment, when the person tells you there is discomfort, release your thumbs and immediately apply the palm of your right hand once again to the affected area, before applying pressure, at the same time as rotating the hand with a clockwise motion. Gradually increase the pressure for a few moments. Release it for a few seconds before applying the pressure again for a further few seconds. It is important to maintain the pressure even when the patient complains of the discomfort. Continue this process; release the pressure and apply it again almost immediately for a further few seconds, before releasing it, and then re-applying the pressure, this time increasing the time to a further five seconds, and then relax.

On the conclusion of the treatment it is important that the person you are treating immediately stands up and walks around the room. Under no circumstances should you allow him or her to remain seated or lying in a horizontal position. Doing so defeats the whole object of the exercise, which is to free the stressed Nadi and ease the inflammation.

Common sense must be used when applying pressure to the painful area. If doing so causes too much discomfort, then stop the treatment until the patient is ready and willing to continue. Under no circumstances must the treatment be carried out if it cause a great deal of discomfort to the patient.

As with all Nadi treatments, on its conclusion the patient should consume a glass of freshly charged water. Remember, pour the water through the air, from one glass to another, until it sparkles and almost comes alive. As I have previously explained, the pouring process encourages the content of prana in the water, making it more invigorating to the cells of the body. The same process can be applied to bath water before you get in it. Using a dish or some other container, scoop the water up into the dish, and allowing it to pass through the air, pour it back into the bath. Do this for several minutes to the entire bath of water, until it seems to come alive. This process of precipitating the Pranic content of bath water has been an extremely effective and integral part of the Yogic method of "Water Therapy" for thousands of years. It invigorates the whole body and encourages relaxation and serenity. It is also an ideal therapy for inflammatory conditions, such as arthritis or rheumatics.

I usually continue the treatment of painful or inflammatory conditions with some Pranic transference. This is the extremely simple and yet effective process involving the precipitation of Prana combined with a little visualization. I have already explained the nature of Prana and how it can be controlled with rhythmic breathing. Prana can also be supported by the imagination which helps to support its effectiveness.

Step 19: Energy transference

Sit the person to be treated on a straight-back chair, making sure that he or she is perfectly relaxed with their eyes closed.

Standing quietly behind them, shake your hands vigorously for two to three minutes, or for as long as you can stand it, until your hands tingle.

With your eyes closed, immediately place a hand on each of the person's shoulders. Inhale a deep breath, and then exhale very slowly, imagining the outpouring breath as powerful rays of blue light.

Once the breath has been fully expelled, vigorously shake your hands again until they tingle, and repeat the process again. In fact, repeat this procedure five or six times, and then relax with your hands on his or her shoulders, and keep them there for five minutes.

On the conclusion of this part of the healing process, repeat the whole procedure again, beginning with shaking your hands, only this time place your hands one either side of the person's head.

As you did previously, inhale a completely breath, and as you breath out, imagine the outpouring breath as being radiant streams of blue light.

Repeat this several times, and then relax with your hands on the person's shoulders. Allow them to remain there for a further five minutes, and then conclude the healing process by allowing the patient to drink some charged water.

With this sort of healing process it is not necessary to actually touch the affected part of the person's body. The holistic action of the treatment encourages the body to heal itself on all levels of existence.

TREATING PAIN WITH PAIN

I have explored the nature of Pranic energy in an earlier chapter and explained how the imagination can be used to infuse it with any colour that you feel is necessary to restore the health and vitality of the body. With the Nadi Technique to physical body is regarded as a sequence of seven colours and their corresponding musical tones. Disease impairs the overall quality of these colours and, as a consequence, causes the tonal effects of the body to go out of tune. When you look upon the human organism in this way, all health conditions become easier to address. The Nadi Technique encourages normality and brings the individual components that make up the whole person harmoniously together once again.

Chapter 11

Colour and you

My wife Dolly has always affirmed that the colours you favour are not necessarily the colours you should always have around you, neither with the clothes you wear, nor in the décor of your home. In fact, in America over the years a study has been made of how colour not only affects us mentally, but also how it somehow affects our physical health and wellbeing. When we are feeling out of sorts and generally under the weather, this is nearly always reflected in the colour of the clothes we choose to wear. Certain personality types often favour particular colours that concur with their personalities. In fact, you frequently see people wearing the same colours all time, and even using these same colours in the décor of their home. People in hot desert climates nearly always wear white garments because of its coolness in the hot and humid atmosphere. In fact, white not only deflects the heat of the sun, but it also deflects negative emotions. Black tends to be quite warm and absorbs the heat of the sun. It also absorbs negative emotions. People who wear black clothes all the time will spend a lot of time in the doldrums and will have some difficulty shaking of depression or feelings of melancholy. The same principles apply to the colour arrangement of your home. A room decorated primarily with varying shades of red will always perpetuate the anxiety levels of an anxious person. Red in the home can also enrage an already fractious person sending him or her into a rage. The colour arrangement of a home has to be carefully thought out, particularly where children are involved. Colours such as red need to be defused with more subtle, complementary colours; colours that don't clash, but subtly blend. Colours really do have a healing effect on a person psychologically speaking, and can either be a joy to live with, or a nightmare to live around. The impact colours in the home have on your psychological status is rarely realized when giving the house a complete makeover. Not only will the wrong colour scheme in the home profoundly affect you psychologically, but its energies will, in time, infiltrate your aura, and in the long term may even impact upon your physical health. The principles of light and colour were in fact known to the ancient Egyptians who used colour to heal diseases of the body and the mind. The colour décor of the home is an extremely important part of the Nadi Technique, as the right colour scheme produces a positive effect upon the tonal effects of the subtle anatomy, encouraging harmony and balance. The same process applies to the colours we actually wear; the wrong colours as much as the right colours, do affect the wearer's personal energy field, causing him or her to either feel depressed or full of the joys of spring, so to speak. It really does make sense when you think about it. Look just how a walk in the countryside raises our spirits and makes us feel so invigorated. In fact, green is the colour of nature; it is a harmonizing colour that stabilizers our emotions and encourages the release of endorphins in the brain, uplifting us and helping us to shake off the blues. The different hues of the many colours of nature, combined with the overall sounds and rhythm of nature itself have a profound effect on the subtle anatomy and thus encourage the precipitation of prana through the network of

Nadis. In years gone by physicians would always recommend that patients recovering from illness should convalesce in a certain place where, they believed, there was "something" in the air that would hasten recovery. Although medical practitioners were most probably not aware of it, this "something" in the air was Prana, the vital force. Prana is prevalent in certain geographical areas, by the sea and also in the countryside. Prana is supported by colour which helps to perpetuate it and making it far more potent. As I have explained in an earlier chapter, although Prana is in the air that we breathe, it is not the air itself. Whilst it is not matter, it is most certainly contained in all forms of matter. The animal and the plant kingdoms take it in with the air, and should Prana not be present with each breath, death would occur. And so we can see that Prana has its own particular parts to play in the manifestation of life, apart from the obvious physiological function. Prana can be effectively charged with colour, as in the case of sending healing to someone at a great distance.

Step 20: Healing yourself with colour

It is a metaphysical fact that the bioluminescence of your personal energy field can become saturated with the vibrations of the various colours that have infiltrated it. As I've previously stated, wearing the same colours all the time, just because you favour those colours, often has an adverse effect on the wearer. The last thing you want to be around when you feel a little depressed or out of sorts, is dark dismal colours, such as black, grey or brown. Colour plays an extremely important psychological part in the day-to-day running of your life, and can even affect your thinking processes Various shades of pink are extremely calming to an anxious mind, and wearing a pink shirt or jumper can encourage serenity and calmness when you're facing a stressful day. Blue is another colour that in itself is healing to someone who is depleted in energy. Students studying for exams will always find it helpful if they wear different shades of blue; indigo will encourage a more focused mind, helping the person to concentrate and retain the information they sufficiently for them to get through his or her exam. There is obviously a little more to this than just throwing on a jumper or shirt. Being aware of the value of colour and how it is able to affect you psychologically and emotionally is a prerequisite to the whole psychological healing process. In the late nineteenth century, a doctor running a sanatorium for people suffering from consumption made a significant discover when treating one of his patients. The man in question had not eaten for days, and it looked to all intents and purposes that he was going to die. All that could now be done for him was to make him as comfortable as possible. His bed was moved to the window so that he could enjoy the strong sunlight streaming through it into the room. He had been there for over an hour when a nurse came to fetch the doctor. Everyone was amazed at the man's remarkable recovery. He was sitting up in bed, bright eyed with colour in his cheeks, asking for something to eat. The doctor in question was puzzled, until it dawned on him that his patient's recovery may well have had something to do with the varying shades of blue glass in the window. He began to experiment with other patients some degree of success. The doctor made an extensive study of the effects of Chrometherapy on the health and well-being of the body, and his studies led him to integrate it into other allopathic treatments. In fact, colour healing was used in ancient Egypt whose practitioners were obviously aware of how powerful the effect of colour was on the body. Although more sophisticated techniques are used today, colour science is still used today, albeit, as a "New Age" therapy.

Step 21: Treating depression

People who suffer with depression frequently see everything as being dark and gloomy, and lifting themselves out of this is nearly always an impossibility. Telling someone who is depressed to pull themselves out of it only makes the sufferer feel worse, as they know full well, if they could pull themselves out of it they would. Colour healing is a complementary therapy and can be used to support the more traditional treatments of allopathic medicine to encourage recovery.

Dark and dismal colours, such as greys, browns and maroons should be avoided, either to wear or in the décor of the home. Instead, pinks, varying shades of blue and the lighter shades of green will produce some remarkable psychological effects on a person suffering with depression. One example of this is the way hospital wards are decorated today as opposed to the 1930s right through to the 1960s and even 1970s. Today there is an understanding of the way colour affects us psychologically, and the way it can either lift us from the doldrums of despair, or pull us further down into an even deeper depression. The right colour arrangements in a hospital ward or bedroom at home, can have a remarkable effect upon a person who is ill, and will aid recovery. As I explained in an earlier chapter, if, as the old saying goes, we can think ourselves into an early grave, then the opposite must also apply—we can surely think ourselves into a healthier longer life. The mind is the common denominator in the whole psychology of wellness, and with the correct attitude to the health of the body, mind and spirit, illness need never be in the equation.

The effects of brighter colours on the mind are nearly always instantaneous, and not just as a psychological placebo effect. Colour works just as effectively on our pets and children, proving that there is far more to colour healing than the mere psychological factors. Try it and see.

When you are feeling depressed or out of sorts, replace the bulb in you sitting room or bedroom with a pink one. Try to eliminate any other light from filtering into the room, and just relax in a comfortable chair for at least an hour. Should you fall asleep, all the better. Repeat this every day and see how better you feel.

Replace the bulb in your bedside light with a pink bulb, and sleep with your head on a pillow covered with a pink pillowslip. Even better, if you can, drape your bed with a pink duvet cover.

Before you go to sleep, sit up in bed for half an hour with the light on. Perhaps you would prefer to read a book or magazine before retiring for the night.

Sleep in this colour ambience every night for a week and see if there is some improvement.

If you are sceptical about colour healing, try it on your dog or cat. Using the same process on your sick or even boisterous pet, you will be amazed just how quickly he or she will respond to the therapy. This should prove to you that a little more than a psychological process is occurring; as your pet has no awareness of these sorts of procedures.

You can experiment with the whole spectrum of colours, treating the condition with the appropriate colour energy. Take a look at the list of colour suggestions below.

RED: Will very often make an anxious person even more anxious. It can make your irritable and angry. But Red will also energize you when you are feeling under the weather or anaemic. When combined with its complementary colour Blue, it is extremely effective in the treatment of addiction to drugs or alcohol. It also encourages clotting to encourage the healing of an open wound.

ORANGE: Will encourage recovery from flu and will maintain balance in the immune system and overall metabolism. Combined with Green it is also a tonic to aid recovery from illness, particularly respiratory conditions.

YELLOW: Will stimulate the endocrine system, and is also a tonic for the kidneys and bladder, as in the case of cystitis and other urinary problems. Combined with Green or Blue it is effective in the treatment of depression or melancholy.

GREEN: Helps to restore balance in the body and encourages the body to heal itself. It is an effective tonic for heart and emotional problems. Combined with Blue it anaesthetizes the body to pain and encourages holistic healing.

BLUE: Produces a calming effect on the body and mind. It is effective in the treatment of any inflammatory or painful diseases. Combined with Purple, it is extremely effective in the treatment of conditions of the nervous system, migraine, cancer and a wide range of other conditions. It will also help to reduce a high temperature.

INDIGO: Encourages sleep and calmness in a restless or anxious mind. It has a holistic effect over the body, and when combined with other relevant colours, it encourages wellness and restores the overall strength and vitality of the body and mind. It can also be used as a general tonic.

VIOLET: Highest colour on the vibratory spectrum. Maybe used in the treatment of cancer and other life-threatening conditions. It complements any other colour increasing their overall strength.

The key word where the use of colour for the treatment of illness is concerned, is *experimentation*, as all colours may be effectively used in various combinations.

One cautionary note: Colour healing may only be used as a complementary therapy, and not to replace allopathic or traditional treatment. Although colour healing is harmless, should you experience any adverse effects, stop the treatment immediately.

Chapter 12

Sex addiction and other hang-ups

Many people mistakenly believe that Yogi Masters advocate the suppression of sex, or even celibacy. Nothing could be further from the truth. On the contrary, the science of Yoga looks upon sex more thoroughly than any other tradition, system or religion. In fact, as well as looking at the physical aspects of the sex act, the science of Yoga also explores the spiritual, emotional and mental aspects of it. In fact, the energies created during sexual activity are closely connected to a potent electromagnetic force located at the base of the spine, known in the science of Yoga as Kundalini. Although Kundalini or "Serpent Fire" as it known in esoteric parlance, is dormant in man, it can be awakened with the use of certain Yogic practices. The arousal of Kundalini encourages the release of incredible powers, known in Yogic tradition as Siddhis, or psychic powers. In fact, Yogi Masters practise certain techniques for directing their sexual energies into subtle, psychic channels, before transmuting them into finer forces. It is their belief that if sexual energies are neither transmuted nor used up in their normal way, their suppression often produces psychological and emotional disorders. It is a fairly known fact that sexual repression often results in sadism, masochism, extreme cruelty and other abnormalities. But this is not meant to be an exploration of the disciplines of Yoga, as much as it is the way sexual frustration affects us psychologically and emotionally.

SEX ADDICTION AND OTHER HANG-UPS

Today it seems to be quite fashionable to be "addicted" to sex, and those who have succumbed to such addiction seek help to deal with it, in the same way that an alcoholic or drug addict would be treated. However, in my opinion the majority of people would be addicted to sex, given half the chance that is. Sex plays an extremely important part of nearly everyone's lives. My own addictions covered an extremely broad spectrum, sex being one of them. I know what I felt like if a week passed by without me having any sexual activity. I became irritable, restless and extremely moody with a short fuse. The key to the whole process of recovery from any addiction, phobia or hang-up, is discipline. When your life is being controlled by any of these, cultivating a more disciplined attitude is extremely difficult but not impossible. Sex is an integral part of life; some people abuse it and will do anything to get it, whilst others treat it as one of life's pleasures, treating it with respect and tenderness. Although I am now a little sceptical about sex addiction, I know from first-hand experience that it can preoccupy your whole life and be the primary focus of everything. I have always had an addictive personality and have always had to be extremely careful not to allow this to go out of control. It was, I suppose, only after many years searching that I discovered the one way of taking complete control of my emotions instead of allowing my emotions to take control of me. Meditation—the key to self-mastery, as we have explored in a previous chapter, is an extremely effective way of gaining control of your life and bringing it back into some semblance of order. As I have already said, what meditation technique suits one person may not necessarily suit another. Some people find it easy to focus the attention for long periods, whilst others have great difficulty in holding the mind steady for even a short time.

This is an extremely simply and yet effective Nadi visualization process that can be used for many different reasons. Unlike other meditation or visualization methods, this exercise needs to be set up before it can be used effectively. Setting it up is perhaps the most difficult part, but once it has been done the whole visualization process requires very little effort.

Step 22: Setting up the exercise

You should sit in a comfortable chair and relax as completely as you can with your eyes closed.

Take a few slow and easy breaths, as we gave done previously, making sure that the inhalations and exhalations are evenly spaced.

Imagine you can see in front of you seven large balloons, each one in a colour of the spectrum.

See each of these balloons floating on the air in front of you, attached to your mind via golden threads.

Spend some time focusing on each balloon until you can see each one very clearly in your mind.

To make the exercise more interesting you might want to give each coloured balloon a funny face. This may help to fix them in your mind more easily.

Before the exercise can be used effectively, you need to spend at least ten minutes (longer if you like) focusing on the coloured balloons, for at least a couple of days, until you are certain you can recall them with some speed and efficiency.

Once you are certain you have the imagery clearly established in your mind, and that you can quickly recall the balloons at a moment's notice, then you are ready to begin the visualization process.

Step 23: The visualization process

Sitting quietly with your eyes closed, breathe rhythmically until the rhythm is fully established in your mind, as before, making certain that the inhalations and exhalations are evenly spaced.

Once you are quite relaxed, mentally create your seven coloured balloons, making sure that they are clearly established on the screen of your mind.

Now, to exert your control over the balloons, one by one let go of each golden thread attached to them, and watch each one floating off into the distance.

Once you have let go of them all, and watched them disappear into the distance, exerting your control over them, gradually bring them back one at a time.

Now that you know that you have control over the balloons, and practise this part of the exercise with little effort, mentally place in each balloon one of the things that are causing you concern, such as an addiction, phobia or hang-up. You can either mentally write whatever it is on an imaginary piece of paper and place it in the balloon, or simply impress the each balloon with your thoughts. Once this has been done, slowly release them again, one at a time, watching them float off towards the distant horizon until they disappear completely.

Once they have gone, bring them back to you once again, one at a time. Repeat this process five times, more if you can, and when you bring them back to you the final time, see the balloons as being empty.

Repeat the same process each day for a week, and on each final time see the balloons as being empty. The imagery is paramount to make the whole mental process effective.

Although quite a laborious process, if you do it correctly, you will be amazed with the psychological effect it will have on the whole of your life. Of course, as with any visualization process of this kind, determination, persistence and the belief that it will work is important.

Addiction to sex, as much as other things, very often leads to anxiety and depression. Both of these conditions are extremely distressing and cause the sufferer very often to be antisocial. This occasionally leads to fear, anger, and overwhelming feelings of guilt, all inwardly directed. When no recognisable situational or psychological based cause can be found, it is sometimes helpful to look toward nutrition for the answer. It has been found that a deficiency in B complex vitamins can in fact lead to various emotional problems. Many physicians have suggested that the diet may play a significant part in hyperactivity, depression and many other behavioural disorders. Nutritional deficiency can be caused by a diet of nutrient-deficient foods, or may even be the result of improper absorption, transport, or metabolism. A balanced diet is essential for the maintenance of the mental as well as the physical health. Exercise helps to control depression, anger and frustrations of all kinds. Regular periods of relaxation, followed by a warm bath, encourages a more serene mind and relaxed body. These are extremely effective treatments to encourage the balance of body, mind and spirit, leading to the control of spontaneous urges and unbridled emotions. More often than not, a person suffering from an anxiety neurosis feels worse in the morning. As I explained in chapter one, this can be the result of hypoglycaemia, low sugar levels in the blood. I remedied this by sucking a glucose tablet, and within moments that overwhelming feeling of panic and shakiness would be gradually eased. I used to take an occasional spoonful of Brewer's yeast in a small glass of orange juice to help with feelings of nervousness. The only things with this is it tends to cause flatulence and makes the urine smell. Apart from those rather unpleasant side-effects, it does help to strengthen and fortify the nervous system in the long term.

Many years ago someone suffering from shock was given a hot drink containing lots of sugar. However, in more recent years it has been suggested that sugar only suffices to increase the amount of adrenalin released into the body, thereby perpetuating the effects of shock. A person in the grip of shock should try and relax as much as possible, with some slow, rhythmic breathing, as we have explored in previous chapters.

Chapter 13

Meditation: the absolute key to freedom

Our emotional, and to some degree, our psychological development, is solely dependent upon our ability to let go of the past. The majority of people have a somewhat morbid preoccupation with the past and seem to delight in re-visiting sad and sometimes hurtful moments of times gone by, thus perpetuating them in their memories. You may very well say that this is human nature, and the whole process of recalling the past is an extremely essential and healthy psychological exercise, and a natural way of dealing negative issues. On one hand, this may very well be the case, at least for a while. On the other hand, when we simply can't let go of events of the past that really disturb us, it prevents us from moving forward, to become stronger and more positive. I am not in any way suggesting that all sad memories are destructive. On the contrary, they can be the building blocks of experience, affording us greater insight into our own lives and allowing us to be able to help others. There are times, in some peoples' lives, when memories are so tainted with negative and disturbing energies that getting on with life is just not an option. Equally, whilst we do need to plan for the future, the future can also present problems, particularly when we constantly worry about something that might happen but more than likely never will. The majority of people worry occasionally about important issues, but it is when that worry becomes the focus of our life that problems arise. Worry impacts upon our physiological and psychological health, and if allowed to persist, will cause stress, anxiety, and in some cases, depression. Worry also affects our posture, breathing and the overall health of our hair, and also causes eruptions to break out on our skin. In other words, worry impairs the overall quality of our health. In fact, the old saying, "it's all in the mind", makes much more sense than we realize. Where our physiological and psychological health is concerned, the mind is truly the common denominator and the overall king of our castle. Meditation not only encourages heightened states of sensory perception, but the whole process of meditation helps us to be more focused and much more able to control negative thinking. In fact, Mindfulness meditation is a process that encourages us to live our lives in the *Now* as opposed to dwelling on the past. Mindfulness as a meditation process is also an ideal psychological tool for de-cluttering the mind and eradicating all unnecessary data. Our parents, for an example, are no doubt unwittingly the architects of our destinies, and from the earliest moments of our life on this planet our future is essentially in their hands. In fact, from a very early age our parents programme us and chastise us by imposing upon us their likes and dislikes, effectively creating us psychologically, emotionally and sometimes spiritually, in their own image, in very much the same way that their parents did to them, and so on through the family history. However, if we are fortunate enough to have well grounded, intelligent and far-seeing parents, then it's a fairly safe bet that you will do well in life, circumstances permitting of course. However, there are other psychological factors to be considered; such as the impressions made on us by our peers and how much we are influenced by the people with whom we associate. We live to all intents and purposes in an extremely competitive world; and a world in which our human frailties and failings are constantly being put to the test, nearly always beyond our endurance. Little wonder then why many of us are insecure and lack confidence. We can't really help but admire those who have done well in life, occasionally to the extent of feeling somewhat jealous, or even resentful. "Good luck to them!" you may very well say, but if you're honest with yourself there is always a part of you that says, "I could have done better than that! If only..." There are many "If onlys" in everyone's life, and there is always a little jealousy when we see others achieve something that inwardly we know we could have done ten times better given the opportunity. But that's just it isn't it? The opportunity is never presented to those who don't expect it! But why do some people who appear to have no real talent get on in life and others with exceptional skills fail in everything they do? Or could it be that those who succeed in life resonate with some sort of universal magnetic force that sets everything in motion for them, affording them success, good health, wealth and happiness? Or is success passed down to us from our forebears, through some sort of genetic electrical impulse system? I would say that there is far more to success than luck or good business acumen, and there is always something a little special about those who succeed that makes them stand out in a crowd. They do say that if you desperately want to succeed in any chosen profession, to the extent that it preoccupies every aspect of your being, then nature will always conspire to lead you into a position whereby your dreams and aspirations may be gratified. Looking at it in this way then we are surely the architects of our own destinies, as long as, that is, we don't allow our parents' control of our minds to impact on us forever, or to interfere with our dreams when we are young! However, as we do not have any say in the matter when we are children, we have to do what we are told, don't we? But in the majority of people there is the potential of a genius that lies dormant, waiting for the moment of arousal. For many that moment never arrives, simply because the dream is never really strong enough. Apart from everything else, Mindfulness meditation encourages the release of the potential we never realized we possessed.

Today meditation is no longer for "certain" kinds of people, and in place of the very often over-prescribed tranquilizers, is even being suggested by many physicians to help with the alleviation of stress and anxiety. As it is now known that meditation lowers stress levels and encourages a more even temperament, it also forms an integral part of the educational curriculum in many schools in India. Research carried out in the University of California into the neurological effects of meditation produced some startling revelations. It was found that meditating regularly produces significant changes in the neurological circuitry of the brain, and in many cases, slightly increases the overall size of the brain itself. Looking at it in this way, meditation is the key to self-mastery, and the way to a long, healthy and happy life.

The Maharishi and TM

I was first introduced to meditation when I attended an introductory talk at a top London hotel in 1966. It was given by the Maharishi Mahesh Yogi, the innovator of Transcendental Meditation, or TM as it became popularly known. The Maharishi's meditation involves the use of a mantra, a word that is personal to the meditator, and which is chanted repeatedly. While TM works for the majority of people, its process is not suitable for some people who find the repetition of a mantra laborious and difficult to maintain. Given that the concentration span and general mental endurance differs from person to person, this is understandable. Bearing this in mind, it is always advisable to experiment with various forms of meditation systems until you find one with which you feel comfortable and that fits perfectly into your daily routine. To the devotee of meditation this may well sound a little paradoxical; as the whole idea of meditation is to discipline and train the mind to focus on one point to the exclusion of everything else. However, in my experience I have found that this only works for a minority, while the majority of those wanting to learn how to meditate need to have a technique that requires little or no effort. In the initial stages, it really doesn't matter what technique of meditation is used, as once the process of meditation has been fully grasped, you can progress to a more complex system.

The objects and use of meditation

Although meditation is today popularly used as a mental process for controlling stress and anxiety, its uses are in fact quite diverse, and cover metaphysical as well as psychological and emotional aspects. In other words, meditation is holistic by its very nature, and once you have formulated an effective working mediation programme, and have begun to practice it religiously each day, positive results will be produced within a very short time.

Karma meditation

Meditation is also an effective way of connecting with the universal mind, (as some refer to it,) as a means of mapping out your destiny and attracting to you the things you desire. Karma meditation is the transcendental process of radically changing your life, by eliminating negative attitudes and making an objective assessment of your life as a whole. This is an extremely effective way of streamlining the way you have allowed yourself to become accustomed to thinking. Karma Meditation is also an effective tool for eradicating habits and putting you in touch with the real essence of your life. A little understanding of the Great Law of Karma will give you a greater insight into what really controls your life, allowing you to see why things have gone wrong, the mistakes you have made and even the right decisions you have taken. Karma Meditation brings about a greater realization of your life, emotionally, psychologically, spiritually and physically. The process is simple and only requires a few minutes of your time.

Three-fold attunement

Three-fold attunement is a system of meditation that initially requires little effort, but then progresses into a more complex process of mental discipline. It consists of three stages: Concentration, Contemplation and finally Meditation, the absolute key to self-mastery. Concentration can be a meditation procedure in itself; so too can contemplation. But when integrated into the Three-Fold system, combined they become one extremely powerful psychological force, and a meditation process that encourages a more positive approach to life in general.

Mindfulness meditation

Although the fundamental principles of Mindfulness have formed the basis for various Buddhist systems of meditation for thousands of years, today this system of meditation has become quite fashionable. Although there are varying approaches to Mindfulness, it basically involves focusing the attention on the present, and giving no space to the past or the future, but just allowing the thoughts to pass through the mind unrestricted. Very little effort is required with this method of meditation to achieve excellent results.

It is important to find the meditation technique that suits you and one you feel comfortable with. I know from years of experience just how beneficial meditation is when integrated into your daily routine. It encourages the development of a peaceful and serene mind, helps to eradicate fears, anxiety and other hang-up, and has a holistic effect upon the practitioner's life. Meditation improves the way you perceive the life around you, giving you a completely different approach to everything, thus lowering stress levels and heightening your awareness of all things. Remember, before you sit for meditation, always spend a few moments relaxing, followed with some slow, rhythmic breathing.

Relaxation

Although I have touched upon relaxation in an earlier chapter, I would like to briefly mention it again. Even if you find meditation is not for you, always spend a little time to relax. This can mean anything from relaxing in the armchair in front of the fire, to taking a leisurely walk in the park or countryside. Whichever you choose, a period of relaxation is essential to dissipate stress and anxiety, and to clear the mind of all the rubbish that you have allowed to accumulate during the course of the day. Stress does not only impact upon our overall health, but it can also cause dermatological eruptions to occur, such as acne, eczema and psoriasis. In some cases it can have a profound effect upon the condition of our hair and even cause it to fall out, as with the condition known as alopecia. So relax and chill out at least once a day. This will add years to your life.

Chapter 14

Getting a grip

As with any substance dependency problem, you have to admit that you have a problem in the first place before it can be treated. Even then, it's still not all that easy addressing it and seeking treatment. Usually, other people see that you've got a problem well before you do. It's the very nature of any addiction to cause the user to be secretive, to lie, and always to make excuses, especially to themselves. It doesn't matter what the addiction is, the mind is always the common denominator, and the sufferer has to somehow find that inner strength to help overcome it. That old and familiar saying "You can take a horse to water, but you can't make it drink" is extremely significant where addiction is concerned. In fact, there are no end of precepts that can be applied to recovery from addiction: "The thousand mile journey begins with the single step." Or, "He who rides the tiger's back must eventually find the courage to dismount." In fact, dealing with any addiction is an extremely lonely and painful process, and although you may have all the support in the world, the struggle is yours alone.

Once the person has faced up to the fact that they do have a problem, and have sought help from the appropriate medical experts, it is important that they stay with it and put themselves completely in their hands. However, both during and after treatment, there are various things that can be carried out to complement treatment. I know from personal experience that there is an extreme emotional aftermath that seems to go on forever. In fact, it will go on forever if you allow it to. Anyone with an addictive nature is always in danger of falling from the wagon, so to speak, and will always be forced to face one temptation after another. In fact, most people with addictive natures often exchange one addiction for another, albeit, a lesser addiction. Dealing with dependency is not easy, as anyone who has been addicted to any form of chemical substances will affirm. Once the problem has been honestly identified, it is important that you apply yourself to the issue in a positive, determined way. Relaxation is important. Not only does this help to reduce anxiety levels, but it also encourages a more focused mind.

I have already explained that the body is permeated by a network of Nadis, transporting Prana from strategic points, known as Chakras, to the organs of the body. In fact, Chakras are connected to the endocrine glands and nerve plexuses, through the Nadi's extensive system, aiding the relentless maintenance of the body's energy levels. When an addiction of any kind is causing major psychological problems, one or more of the Chakras are either spiralling almost out of control, or are extremely sluggish. Before treatment commences, it needs to be determined which chakras have been affected.

Step 24: Dowsing the chakras

For this you will need a pendulum and the cooperation of a friend. You will also need a notepad and pen and one moderately powerful metal magnet.

If you are being treated, you should lie in a horizontal position, either on the floor or bed. If you are treating someone else, they should assume the same position.

Taking the pendulum in one hand, hold it as close to the person's forehead as possible, making a note of the rotational direction of the pendulum, clockwise or anticlockwise.

Move down to the area of the throat, again making a note of the pendulum's movement. As the location of each individual's chakras vary from person to person, you may find it necessary to move the pendulum around the area until the vortex is found. The chakras are not always located in the places specified on a chart.

Repeat the same process with each chakra, and once the area of the base chakra is reached, follow the same route back up the body, concluding with brow centre.

Wait a few minutes before repeating the whole process again. This is carried out to make sure the chakra calculations have not changed.

You may notice that some chakras produce very little movement in the pendulum, while others cause it to swing erratically. Once the sluggish chakras have been treated, the other chakras will normalize automatically.

Treatment

The person should now lie on his or her tummy with their arms pulled into their sides. Make they are quite comfortable, as this would only defeat the whole object of the exercise. Avoid this treatment if the person has a pacemaker fitted.

Take the magnet in the left hand, and holding it as close to the back of the person's head without touching it, slowly move it in a clockwise manner, down his or her back, stopping at the base of the spine. Still rotating the magnet with a clockwise motion, hold it there for a minute or so, before repeating the same process, back along the spine, concluding the treatment at the back of the person's head.

Still rotating the magnet with a clockwise motions, hold it there for a further minute before relaxing.

The whole thing should now be concluded with the rotating hands treatment given in an earlier chapter. Just reiterate this: Place your left hand as close to the back of the person's head as possible, without touching it. Begin the treatment by rotating your left hand with a clockwise motion, and with the right hand placed over the left hand, without touching it, rotate that one with an anticlockwise motion. Once you have mastered this process, slowly move the rotating hands simultaneously from the person's head, along the spine, concluding the rotating treatment at the base of the spine.

Still simultaneously rotating the hands, allow them to remain there for a minutes, before following the same procedure back along the spine, concluding the treatment at the back of the head.

Finally, with the fingers of both hands spread apart, for a further two minutes or so, make quick, random sweeping passes across the person's body, again without actually touching it.

I have explained earlier that the human form is an electro-magnetic unit of incredible power; this being the case, the metal magnets create a resonance with the person's energy field, encourage a more even flow of energy through the individual chakras. The treatment may have to be applied a few times to achieve positive results. The only way you will be able to determine if the treatment has been successful is to dowse the individual chakras to see if the polarity has changed. Technically, the rotational movements of the chakras should alternate clockwise, anticlockwise, clockwise and so on. However, because of the stresses and chores of the day, this is rarely seen. The brow chakra of a male should have a clockwise rotation, the throat chakra anticlockwise, the heart chakra clockwise, so on and so forth. Whilst in the female the chakras rotate the opposite way round. The brow chakra anticlockwise, the throat chakra clockwise, and so on.

The central spinal Nadi, Sushumna, is an extremely important channel, as it is this one that supports and controls the movement of another powerful energy called Kundalini. Although there are more specific meditation techniques to precipitate the movement of this force, this is a completely specialized subject and not relevant to this system of healing. Nonetheless, I will give you a brief explanation as to the nature of Kundalini. The concept of a key universal energy that can be activated in the body and controlled by meditation is, in fact, found in a number of esoteric traditions. Kundalini is a concentration of cosmic life energy, dormant at the base of the spine and coiled two and a half times like a serpent. The mouth of this serpent appears to be closed around the base chakra, Muladhara. Once the individual chakras have been treated, to ensure the transition of energy is maintained along the Nadis, you will find the following treatment extremely effective.

Step 25: Spinal manipulation

The person being treated should lie face down, with his or her hands by their sides. A light, loose-fitting garment should be worn.

GETTING A GRIP

The person carrying out the treatment should use the fingers of both hands to gently massage the back of the person's neck. Maintain this for one minute.

Next, move the fingers slightly down the spine, to the base of the neck, with the index fingers on one side of the spine, and the thumbs on the other, gently manipulate that area for a few moments, before slowly moving down a further four inches down the spine.

Maintain the movement of the fingers and thumbs, spending no more than thirty seconds at each point, and following a straight route down the whole of the spine.

When the coccyx is reached, with the fingers of both hands stretched outward, making sweeping passes from the base of the spine to the back of the person's head. At which point, both hands should rest for thirty seconds, one on top of the other, on the back of the person's head.

Repeat the whole process two more times, always concluding with both hands resting on the back of the person's head.

Although not absolutely necessary, sometimes this exercise benefits from a little visualization, with the fingers and thumbs manipulating intense white light along the person's spine. Also, should you be well acquainted with the person you are treating (or who is treating you, as in partner or family member) the treatment is best carried out against the person's bare flesh. Contact in this way facilitates the prana more efficiently down the primary Nadi. After receiving this treatment it is usual to feel quite tired, and so I always suggest a period of rest. As always, on the conclusion of the treatment, drink a glass of charged water. Always charge the water using the same pouring process. Pour it through the air, from one glass to another, until the water sparkles and seems to come alive.

Chapter 15

Restless and insomnia

If you are one of those people who falls asleep as soon as your head touches the pillow, then you are extremely fortunate. However, many people have difficulty getting to sleep, and find that when they climb into bed, even though their body is extremely tired, their mind carries on replaying the events of the day. Even after a hard day at work, some people still have difficulty falling asleep, and find to impossible to stop the mind from wandering from one thing to another. The Nadi Technique for quietening a restless mind at night addresses the problem simply and effectively by looking at the cause and curing it. The inability to sleep, even when you are extremely tired, can be caused by many different things, one of which is the magnetic pull of the planets, particularly the moon, on the earth. Moving the position of the bed is the first thing you must try so that your feet point towards the south and your head towards the north. This one simple thing nearly always solves the problem of insomnia and restlessness. A sceptic may very well dismiss this suggestion, but the truth is, the magnetic pull of the moon on the earth causes many neurological disturbances than you might imagine. Besides, you've got nothing at all to lose and everything to gain.

Should you be in the habit of eating a large meal late at night, then that must also be changed. If you simply must eat before going to bed, eat a light meal at least two or three hours before you retire; this is much easier on the digestion and will not disturb your sleep pattern and will encourage a more restful night.

If it's just not possible to sleep in a totally dark room, then wear a blindfold to block out any light. This will cut-out any stimulating distractions and encourage more restful sleep.

Make sure that the room is well ventilated. Poor ventilation also contributes to the inability to sleep.

Never sleep with your arms under your head. Arms raised above your head when you are trying to sleep causes tension, and in the morning you will feel as though you haven't slept at all.

Try to avoid staying up late. The best and most rested sleep is the one before midnight.

Whenever possible, try to sleep without wearing any night attire, so as to allow the skin to breathe freely.

Never keep plants or flowers in the bedroom at night.

In bed do not sleep with your head raised too high and try to keep the spine as straight as possible.

Before retiring avoid stimulating beverages such as tea, coffee or alcohol.

Finally, before retiring follow the rhythmic breathing procedure given in an earlier chapter. Slow rhythmic breathing makes the mind quiet and relaxes the whole body in preparation for sleep.

Controlling the inflowing prana with rhythmic breathing encourages the equilibrium of body, mind and spirit, and also maintains the overall health of the body. It enriches all the organs of the body by infusing them with vitality. In fact, breath is life, life is solely dependent upon breath. The process of respiration is paramount in cell reproduction and ensures that our life-giving blood is infused with Pranic energy. Rhythmic breathing maintains balance in the body and helps to maintain a healthy heart. One particular Pranic stimulating exercise is excellent for affecting the circulation in the lungs and improving the intake of oxygen.

Step 26: Lung and heart stimulation

Stand up straight and raise your right hand as high as you can above your head.

Slowly breathe-in, and when the breath is complete, hold it for a count of four.

Breathe-out slowly, expelling all the air from your lungs, and as you do so, push up standing on your toes, stretching your arm even higher. Then relax with your arm by your side.

Repeat the process with the same arm two more times. Then relax.

Almost immediately, raise your left arm and repeat the exercise. Slowly breathe-in. When the breath is complete, hold it for the count of four, and then as you breathe-out, reach up even higher, standing on your toes and stretching your arm as high as you can. Now relax.

Repeat the same process with the left arm two more times, and then relax.

This Pranic exercise is an excellent tonic either to begin the day, or to prepare for the night. It rejuvenates the brain, heart and central nervous system and encourages the mind to be more focused and alert. Do not practise this exercise more than the suggested amount of times, as this may well defeat the whole object of the exercise.

Step 27: Encouraging restfulness

Lie on your bed and relax the body as much as you possibly.

Breathe rhythmically for a few moments, making sure that the inhalations and exhalations are evenly spaced.

Place the index finger and middle fingers of both hands on the centre of the forehead, with the middle fingers touching, and apply a little pressure as you do so.

Slowly breathe-in, whilst simultaneously pulling the fingers slightly upward, drawing the surface of the skin of the forehead as you do so, and holding the fingers in that position, along with breath retention for the count of four. Maintain the slight pressure as you do so.

Exhale, expelling as much of the air from your lungs as possible, whilst simultaneously allowing the fingers to draw down the skin to its original position, maintaining a slight pressure as you do so.

Repeat the whole process for or five times, before relaxing.

As well as encouraging a restful sleep, this process will also relieve tension and any discomfort it causes. It can also be applied during the day, particularly if your work involves sitting in front of a computer.

You will recall that I explained in an earlier chapter, that Prana is constantly being conveyed along the Nadis in the relentless process of maintaining balance in the body. For many different reasons, the flow of Prana is sometimes inhibited, thus affecting the corresponding part of the body. Although a visit to an acupuncturist or reflexologist nearly always directly addresses the problem, with the exercises given in this book, you can easily deal with the problem yourself. After all, protection is far better than cure, wouldn't you say. When practising rhythmic breathing, never strain your breathing or make it a labour. Also, try to vary

100

the pace of your rhythmic breathing, occasionally making the exhalations of breath marginally longer than the inhalations. The exhalations are sometimes more important as they help to improve the elasticity of the lungs, thereby encouraging a greater lung capacity. The physiological effects of rhythmic breathing cover a broad spectrum, and also help to build more red blood cells. I have stated in an earlier chapter that, because of the way we are taught at school when we are young, the way we breathe in the Western world is inefficient. Incorrect breathing causes bad posture and comprises our respiratory system, which in turn impacts our emotional and psychological states. Correct breathing encourages the development of streamlined thinking processes, and also supports a more efficient assimilation of oxygen in our bodies. It also lessens infections and adds years to our lives. The Nadi Technique considers all alternative routes, and is an extremely effective way of energizing the body to improve the overall health and vitality.

Chapter 16

Overview of healing

As well as using the Nadi Technique to treat your own health issues, combined with a variety of other spiritual and psychic healing methods, it can also be used to treat the health conditions of other people. Although true spiritual healing does not require the person who is being treated to have faith or belief in it, when using the Nadi Technique the healing practitioner does need to have a certain amount of compassion in order to facilitate the healing process. Although the healing process will still produce a noticeable effect, without empathy results may not be as spontaneous or as long-lasting. Many healing practitioners will most probably totally disagree with this statement, but I am writing purely on my own experiences and the many observations I have made over the years. The Nadi Technique explores and includes numerous methods of healing, some of which have been mentioned in an earlier chapter. However, all Nadi methods are applied to precipitate the movement of Prana in the body and to energize it, thus encouraging the self-healing process. When the Nadi Technique is frequently applied, balance is maintained in the body and it then learns to heal itself. This process may either be carried out through touch or with simple mental imagery techniques. Experimentation is paramount to see which methods work for you. Many practitioners of the Nadi Technique find it helpful to modify some of the treatments to suit the way they work. As long as the fundamental principles of the Nadi Technique are kept, modifying them to format your own system is totally acceptable. There is also an extremely powerful psychology underlying the process of the Nadi healing Technique, whether applied to oneself or administered to someone else. The discomfort of a child who bangs its head, or bruises its knee is easily relieved with the rub of a mother's hand and a few calming words, "There, mummy's made it better." With the pain gone, and the tears dried, the child carries on playing, completely forgetting the discomfort of his or her little mishap. The soothing and reassuring hand of our loved one on our forehead when we are feeling poorly, comforts us and quickly sends us to sleep. When we have a headache we instinctively apply a little pressure to the painful area to obtain relief. So there is most definitely something quite special in the human touch that is able to ease pain and even cure disease. Of course, easing the discomfort of a headache is one thing, but curing disease is something quite different altogether. Healing has always been an integral part of human life; from the biblical accounts of the healings of Jesus, to even the unorthodox healing practices of Rasputin, the so-called "Mad Monk". The whole healing system of the Nadi Technique is about gaining control of your body and mind and maintaining the health of both. Some of the self-healing methods may not work for you, whilst others will prove extremely effective.

Although the Nadi Technique is not in any way dependent on faith, when the healing process is applied with a strong sense of compassion, the energy created with this is transferred to the person receiving the treatment. Compassion with the overwhelming intention to relieve the pain and discomfort, culminates into an extremely powerful holistic healing force that can produce remarkable results. Unlike the process of spiritual healing, the Nadi Technique can be applied by anyone with an interest in holistic healing. Spiritual healing is a completely different process and really does require a great deal of development. In my opinion not everyone possesses the potential to develop a healing ability, nor does the desire to be a healer mean that you are one. Spiritual healing is quite specific, and the ability to heal more often than not occurs quite spontaneously, and although not in all cases, it sometimes develops as a result of the person's own experience with serious illness. It is through this sort of experience that prana is spontaneously transported along the Nadis, thus causing activation of the appropriate chakras.

Healing in one form or another has been practised from time immemorial. Up until as late as the eighteenth century in Britain, some people believed that the monarch's so-called "Royal Touch" could cure all manner of ailments, and would go to any lengths to be touched by the King or Queen. Today it is a well-known scientific face that touching does have specific therapeutic value, particularly in relieving pain. Scientists in fact believe that stimulation of the nerves through the process of touching or rubbing interrupts the signals received by the neurological pain receptors, thus alleviating the full sensation of pain impulses on the brain's cerebral cortex. Of course, this does not explain why some people possess the ability to ease discomfort and pain in another person, and some do not. Some healing practitioners somehow discharge a very subtle energy that can affect the neurological circuitry of a person who is unwell or simply out of sorts, promoting feelings of calmness and well-being.

OVERVIEW OF HEALING

It may well come as a great surprise to many people to learn that all diseases do have their own particular odours, and many doctors rely on their sense of smell as a diagnostic tool. In fact, many medical practitioners become accustomed to the actual smell of disease, and are able to make a diagnosis by simply identifying a specific odour. Although healing practitioners should never offer a diagnosis for a health condition, unless medically qualified of course, the ability to actually identify a health condition through the sense of smell is extremely useful. When regularly treating disease of any kind, identifying disease through its odour frequently develops. The Nadi Technique encourages the development of the practitioner's sensitivity, so that he or she finds it easy to become attuned to the person they are treating. It is believed that certain diseases do have distinctive odours, caused by a change in the metabolic processes associated with the patient's condition. Victorian doctors were very often able to identify arsenic poisoning because of the odour of garlic. A fruity smell on the breath would be an indication that either the person was diabetic or starving. Some illnesses possess some very distinctive odours and may easily be identified. For example, German Measles apparently smells like plucked feathers; Scrofula, which is a form of tuberculosis, smells like stale beer. Typhoid has the distinctive smell of baking bread, and Yellow Fever has the overwhelming smell of a butcher's shop. An experienced surgeon will always be able to identify bacterial infection by the smell of the patient's bandages. A musty, damp cellar smell can be an indication of an infected wound. The breath of a person in a diabetic coma has an acetone smell, or smells like Pear Drops. Experience alone will encourage the development of your sense of "smell" when administering

105

healing, and although in time the different odours of illness will not be as apparent to you, they will still influence your senses and continue to intuitively guide you. It is a well-known psychological fact that obnoxious smells become less noticeable in time, especially when you are frequently exposed to them. Even though this is the case your ability to instinctively sense disease through odour will continue to develop. The ability to smell disease is extremely useful when applying the Nadi Technique to someone who is unwell. It will help you to understand where exactly the treatment needs to be applied. Even though the Nadi Technique is a holistic process, occasionally it is more beneficial to apply it directly to the affected part of the body. Of course, as this book is about you, and the ability to correct your own imbalances, this sort of treatment could only be used when you are applying to someone else. The Nadi Technique corrects any imbalances in the body, simply by precipitating the inhibited flow of Prana through the Nadis. Working on the premise that the root course of illness is in the mind, this being the common denominator, and ruler of the kingdom of cells. I have stated in a previous chapter that, in our study of the effects of the Nadi Technique on the human organism, it must be borne in mind that before we can heal the part it is necessary to first consider the *whole*. This is the fundamental principle underlying the holistic healing process of the Nadi Technique. I have already explained the importance of the chakra system and how these are connected to the endocrine glands and nerve plexuses, supported by the extensive system of Nadis, along which Prana is conveyed, from the chakras to the organs of the physical body, in the relentless process of maintaining the overall health and balance of the body. In the next chapter we will explore the importance of the endocrine system and the part it plays in the smooth running of the body's health and equilibrium.

Chapter 17

The science of the endocrine system

The efficiency of the body as a whole is to all intents and purposes dependent upon the individual components of which the whole unit is comprised. Should a single part of the body cease to function effectively, then the efficiency of the whole unit would be greatly impaired as a direct consequence.

The endocrine glands play an extremely important part in the holistic health of the body, and the overall personality is to some extent regulated by one or the other of these glands.

The endocrine glands are sometimes referred to as "ductless" because they have no ducts and secrete their hormones directly into the bloodstream. These glands in fact collectively form the so-called endocrine system which directly corresponds with the chakra system, and vice versa. As I have already said, the overall health of the body is dependent upon the efficiency of the endocrine glands, and the inefficiency of one of the glands will impact upon the others.

The endocrine system is comprised of the pineal and the pituitary glands, located strategically in the cavity of the skull; the thyroid and parathyroid, situated near the larynx at the base of the neck; the thymus, situated strategically in the chest above the heart; the pair of adrenals (or suprarenals) topping the kidneys almost like tiny hoods; the gonads of the male and female reproductive system. All the endocrine glands are closely related and supplement and depend upon each other. The healthy functioning of the endocrine glands is of paramount importance to the well-being of the individual, and the minute secretions of hormones from each are responsible for the development of the genius as opposed to the imbecile, or the restricted growth of the dwarf as opposed to the giant, or even the release of either happiness as opposed to sadness. In fact, the endocrine glands exert an incredible influence over the growth of our bodies and the development of the working of our minds, and in more ways than one really make us who and what we are. Their persuasive influence affects everything we do, and not only helps to determine the shape of our body, but also affects the way we think and behave.

The pituitary gland is very often perceived as the most important gland, and has been described as the gland that "gives the tune to all other glands", which appear to be totally dependent on it. In fact, the pituitary gland encourages and controls the inner mobility and efficiency of the whole system and promotes and controls the growth of the body, glands and organs including sexual development. It supervises and maintains the efficient performance of the various structures and helps in the prevention of excessive fat accumulation. A happy uncomplicated individual without any hang-ups is nearly always indicative of a healthy, active and normal working pituitary gland.

The pineal gland is a pine-shaped body deep within the brain. This is usually larger in a child than in an adult, and marginally more developed in a female than in a male. The pineal gland appears to harmonize the internal environment, and supervises the development of the other glands, thus maintaining their synchronicity and polarity in relation to each other. The pathological condition of the pineal gland is believed to exert a strong influence over the sex glands and causes the premature development of the system as a whole. In the pineal gland's normal condition it promotes harmony and efficient functioning of the endocrine system.

The inner activity of the endocrine system is controlled by the thyroid gland, ensuring that the tissues are fully active with no water retention, and that there is no densification of bones. The general condition of the thyroid is responsible for whether a person is very active or lethargic, tired or energetic, alert or depressed. The thyroid also controls the development and function of the sex organs.

The overall stability of the functioning within our body is to some extent influenced by the parathyroid glands, which maintains metabolic equilibrium by supervising the distribution and activity of calcium and phosphorus in our system. The healthy performance of these glands maintains constant balance of calcium and phosphorus, resulting in poise and tranquillity.

When puberty is reached the actual size and importance of the thymus gland is reduced, as the part it previously played supervising natural growth and development should have by then been successfully achieved. The shrinking process of the thymus gland ensures that the natural adjustment of the individual is not impaired in anyway whatsoever.

The inner vitality and energy is encouraged by the adrenal glands, with a relentless drive to action, perception, activity, courage and vigour. The adrenal glands encourage oxygenation of the bloodstream, intensifying this process with revitalized power.

THE SCIENCE OF THE ENDOCRINE SYSTEM

The phenomenon of attraction to the opposite sex is largely the result of healthy gonads of the male and female reproductive system, whose primary function is to maintain that attraction by encouraging the personality to radiate with confidence and self-assurance. The release of hormones from the gonads encourages inner warmth in the system ensuring that flexibility is maintained and that the overall health and vitality continues.

The overall health and vitality of the endocrine system is to some extent maintained by the regular distribution of the life force—Prana—throughout the entire organism. A little understanding of the way in which this life force permeates the subtle channels should enable every Nadi practitioner to more effectively supervise the healing treatment, and thus facilitate the whole Nadi process more efficiently.

As well as a healthy diet, preferably meat-free, it is vitally important to hydrate the body well. To precipitate the levels of Prana in the water you drink, as I have explained in previous chapters, it should be poured several times through the air, from one glass to another, until the water appears to almost sparkle with vitality. The whole glass should be consumed, especially after a treatment has been applied. Should a non-meat diet not appeal to you, eat as much vegetables and fruit as you can, making sure that you slowly masticate what you eat, thus ensuring all the health-giving properties are taken into the stomach.

Today it is common knowledge that stress, worry and anxiety are contributory factors for many diseases. I have said elsewhere that the mind is most certainly the common denominator; it can, as the saying goes, put you into an early grave. If that is true, then the opposite must also apply. With the correct mental attitude,

111

one can promote good health, vitality and harmony. Apart from all the other treatments, the Nadi Technique also teaches "Mind Balancing" and healing the body through suggestion. In the following chapter we will explore the concept of healing the body with the mind.

Chapter 18

Healing with the mind: suggestion

All the components that make up the whole body are to some extent controlled by the mind. In fact the processes of *thought* greatly influence the way we feel on a day to day basis. One example is when we are afraid or anxious; the physiological effects become extremely apparent. We perspire, the heart races, and our hands shake, all in response to the signals sent to the body from the mind, the central control system. A similar physiological process occurs when we are happy or excited about something. We feel a rush of adrenalin, the heart quickens and our face glows. The endorphins released into the bloodstream make us feel good. It makes sense then, that if the mind can exert such a powerful influence over the body, then the same mental power may be used to promote well-being and even cure disease. Of course, depression is something else altogether. Depression is insidious and can occur for many different reasons, chemical imbalance being one such cause, a neurological circuitry malfunction probably another. Even emotional trauma can cause depression, as well as the loss of a loved one. When you are depressed thinking in a positive way is impossible. None-the-less, using the mind to heal the body is more than a possibility. It is called suggestive healing, a method of persuaded all the components of the body to join forces to gather sufficient strength to heal itself. First of all, the force of suggestive healing becomes greater with more intensity with repetition. It works on the same principle as the repetition of a mantra to produce a calming effect upon the mind. As well as treating yourself with suggestive healing, the same process can be applied to heal someone else. However, it needs to be repetitively consistent and carried out daily until positive results are experienced. The process is simple. First of all, let's explore the process of suggestive healing when applied to one's self.

Step 28: Suggestive process

You must carry out the treatment in a calm place and at a time when you know you will not be disturbed. I always equate suggestive healing to an army attacking the enemy. The attack has to be carried out from all sides, repetitively, systematically and relentlessly. The suggestion needs to fill your mind so that it is quickly absorbed by the subconscious mind. The exercise relies totally on your visualization skill, and comes in two parts. The first part is a cleansing process. Remember not to allow your concentration to drift, even for one second, from the visualization imagery, as this would merely defeat the whole object of the exercise.

Process 1

With your eyes closed, breathe rhythmically until the rhythm of your breathing is fully established and your mind is quiet and the body relaxed.

Focus your full attention on your breathing, and with each inhalation see a stream of intense white light being drawn into your body.

114

Hold the breath for the count of four, while mentally watching this intense white light circulating your entire body.

Forcibly exhale through your mouth, seeing the breath as a grey or even black discharge, issuing forth with the exhaled breath.

Repeat this process three times, and then relax for a few moments before moving to the next process.

Process 2

For this part of the process you will need to mentally scan your whole body, seeing the individual components, as best as you can, the heart, lungs, liver and stomach. Don't worry too much if the organs are not in perfect anatomical order, as the power created by your mind will locate them during the exercise. But be forcible, positive and determined.

First of all, mentally speak to your heart as you would an old friend. Persuade it to be healthy, and to beat regularly and in harmony with the rest of its companions. Tell it to take control and to keep order. This powerful organ regulates everything and maintains order in the body.

Now, speak to your liver with the same persuasive attitude. Order it to perform the duty of purifying the toxins and maintain the health of the bloodstream and keep everything balanced. Be persistent, and try to visualize the liver as you speak.

Now, follow this by visualizing your stomach and the digestive organs, instructing them to function well and to take care of the relentless processing of the food you eat. Ask it to stay healthy and always efficiently assimilate the nutrients so that your digestion always functions properly with no problems.

115

Next, focus your attention on your lungs, breathing-in and out with a nice gentle rhythm, mentally instructing them to function effectively, free from infection, and always allowing Prana the life-force to be circulated efficiently through the body, maintaining the health, vitality and equilibrium of the whole body.

Finally, express your sincere appreciation to all the organs of the body for their help in maintaining your health, asking them to continue to do so, thus ensuring you a long and healthy life.

Should you be sceptical about this process of self-healing, it will not work for you. You really do have to believe in suggestive healing, and know that it will work if applied in a positive, consistent way. The cultivation of positive thinking is paramount when applying healing to yourself. I am always reminded of the ancient precept: "As a man thinketh in his heart, so is he." Apart from all the practical applications integrated into the self-healing process of the Nadi Technique, it also encourages a more positive way of thinking, plus a complete change in attitude towards everything. Suggestive healing may also be applied to another person using the same process.

Here's what to do

The person may either lie in a horizontal position, or relax in a comfortable chair, whichever he or she prefers.

Talk him or her through the relaxation process in a reassuring voice, explaining how to breathe rhythmically, thus ensuring they feel relaxed.

Make them aware of the various components of their body, talking them through the various organs, before finally getting them to focus their attention on the heart.

116

HEALING WITH THE MIND: SUGGESTION

As with the previous treatment, as the person to spend a few moments mentally persuading their heart to beat with a regular rhythm, and always to maintain a healthy function, ensuring that all the other bodily components work in harmony with each other.

Now, as you did previously, talk the person through to the liver, instructing them to mentally persuade it to efficiently perform the function of eradicating all the toxins from the blood stream, ensuring the maintenance of all the other organs.

It is important for you to occasionally interject reassuring dialogue, encouraging them to follow the same process of treating all the organs of their body as intelligent units, individual, and yet collectively working as one whole. Once the person has mastered the process of using visualization and suggestion to influence the organs of the body, then should begin to see positive results. For the healing process to be successful, visualization is paramount. The whole process should be consistent and the mind should not be allowed to wander even for a second.

Chapter 19

Be positive and in tune with the universe

It is really not all that easy to transform the conditioning of a lifetime, into a new and more dynamic way of thinking about yourself and everything else around you. If, like me, you were sheltered and mollycoddled as a child, you probably suffer with all the insecurities and hang-ups that I had to cope with in my young adult life. So you will appreciate exactly how difficult it makes life, particularly when you desperately want to be like the majority of so-called "normal" people your age. Converting your insecurities into positive and confident energies is an absolutely arduous task, but believe me, it is not impossible. I have always equated the initial stages of the process with the various parts actors play on the stage. They put themselves totally into the character they are playing, and completely take-over the personality of that character, to the extent that they become that person completely. When the production has finished, it more than likely takes the actor some time to get the character completely out of his or her head. Depending on the theme of the play, and the nature of the character the actor has been playing, they can be affected emotionally, at least for a short while. As the title of this books suggests, we do have to get a grip and take control of our lives, instead of allowing our life to take control of us. I know you are probably thinking "this is easier said than done!" But, the truth is, it's either make every effort to do this, or live a life of veritable misery and be subservient to other people. You do have to face your demons head on, and only then will they turn and run from you. I've already spoken in an earlier chapter about aversion therapy; that is facing your fears instead of running from them. Once you have managed to do that, there's still a lot of work to do on yourself. There are two Sanskrit words in yoga, *YAMA* and *NYAMA*. Yama means avoidance of destruction, injury, envy, untruth, dishonesty and much more. Nyama basically means internal and external purification, contentment, strength of character, patience, calmness of mind, kindness and charity. It is a good idea to make an extensive study of these two words and endeavour to fix the meanings of each in your mind. Contemplate their meaning and how they can each be applied to your life. For example, with Yama and avoidance: avoid self-pity, over-indulgence, and anger. In fact avoid all the things that hinder your progress and positivity. Be honest with yourself as you mentally make a detailed analysis of Yama and all the things it suggests. Spend some time on the word itself, so that you full understand its meaning and the implications of all the negative aspects connected to it.

Explore the word Nyama and all that it implies. For example, what does internal and external purification mean to you? If it makes it easier for you, make a note of everything in a personal notebook, so that you can refer to it when you need to. The two words need to be fixed firmly and positively in your mind, so that they almost become your personal mantras. Make a detailed study of all the things connected to the words and make every effort to address them as best and as systematically as you can. Pay particular attention to Nyama and calmness of mind. Each time you are faced with a difficult situation and one that makes you anxious or depressed, refer to Nyama, and then re-inspect its meaning. This in itself will bring you some solace and peace of mind. Contemplating on these two words must be carried out every day, systematically and relentlessly, if they are to successfully work for you.

Step 29: Transforming the way you think

First of all, you need to have the correct intention and really and truly want to move forward. Regardless of whether or not you have never had a positive approach to your life, it is never too late to change the way you think. Find a quiet moment and relax. It's time to make a plan, and stick to it.

Contemplation planning and focus

Never just sit back and expect your circumstances and mental attitude to change by themselves. Although it's good to have the support of family and friends, try not to rely on other people. You know the old saying, you can give a man fish every day of his life, but if you give him a fishing rod and teach him how to fish, he can feed himself. Take a quiet moment and use it wisely. In your quiet moment you need to focus your attention on all the things you would like to change in your life, mentally seeing yourself as the person you would really like to be.

Avoid admiring other people, and do not compare yourself to anyone.

Make a detailed analysis of yourself, and try to take an objective look at your faults; weaknesses, phobias, anxieties and dependencies. It helps if you sit comfortably with a hand-held mirror so that you can study your reflection. Make a study of your features and see just how unique you are. If you've never liked the

120

way you look, remember, that's just your own opinion. Other people will see a very "different" you.

Make a detailed analysis of the things that cause your hang-ups, and make every effort to see them for what they are, self-destructive and a hindrance, and bearing no connection to reality.

Breathe rhythmically for a few moments until the rhythm is fully established, and contemplate your connection with the universe.

Try to see yourself objectively as other people see you, making a note of all the things you would change about yourself. Having done this, sit quietly reading through the list, and try to be as honest with yourself as you can. Do you really and truly dislike yourself? With your eyes closed, repeat several times, "I am a nice person. I am a nice person. I am a very nice person." And so on.

Think about what you are saying and allow your words to become your affirmations. Repeat these words every day, even twice a day. Integrate this part into your daily programme until you believe what you are saying. Your subconscious mind will eventually take what you are telling it on board. Give it time.

Universal resonance

The energies you have become accustomed to creating through negative thinking will have resonated with the universe and pulled you further into a negative state of mind. In fact, the universe will always work with you, regardless of whether you think positive or negative thoughts. A little understanding of the Great Law of Attraction, will help you to take control of your own life. I have said elsewhere in this books that you are the architect of your own destiny simply by the way you think; and you are constantly peopling your own private portion of space with the thoughts you release. In other words, the universe will always conspire to lead you into the appropriate situation in which your thoughts can be gratified. It makes sense then that the opposite also applies. The fundamental principles of the Great Law of Attraction mean that you are always in control of your own destiny, and really do have the power to transform your life at any time. Your body is subservient to your mind and obeys its every command. When the mind sinks into a negative, darker state, the body responds in sympathy, falling into illness or even disease. If you persist with such negative thinking, the universe will quickly harmonize with the thoughts you release. The health of the body, as well as the circumstances of your life, are more or less created by the way you have become accustomed to thinking. Thoughts of fear have the power to kill you almost as quickly as a bullet. On the other hand, brighter and more positive thoughts quickly streamline your life, encouraging good health and success. You should meditate on these facts for at least ten minutes every day. Before you begin, always sit quietly in a contemplative state for ten minutes, during which you should make a mental connection with the universal mind, at the same time as sending out the request for the things you require to make you positive, charismatic, healthy, happy and wise. Do not send out your request feebly, but send it out forcibly and with confidence, almost as though you are in a marketplace making a purchase for something that you need. Then in your meditative moment, again sitting quietly, do all that you can to make the mind blank. When thoughts, images or ideas pass through your mind, try not to retain them; allow them to pass freely. Focus your attention on your breathing, making sure that the inhalations and exhalations are evenly spaced. Maintain this state of mind for ten minutes, longer if you feel comfortable.

Remember, focus all your attention on the preceding contemplative state, making sure that the imagery is extremely vivid. If you can, try to make the things you are requesting as vivid and clear as though you already possessed them. In the initial stages of this exercise you may have some difficulty doing this, but in time it will become almost second nature.

As the human organism is a unit of incredible power, and a network of channels; one of the ways to ensure that energy flows freely is to tap the channels at strategic points. Accompanying this tapping with simple affirmations encourages a more powerful force to precipitate the mobility of the energy. In the following chapter we will explore this process more.

Chapter 20

Tapping to release negative emotions

You most probably understand by now that the Nadi Technique is all about energizing the body with the intention of curing, or at least alleviating health issues. The curing of low self-esteem and other psychological or emotional issues, can be effectively carried out with simple tapping techniques. Although "Tapping" as an alternative therapy is quite popular today, there are other methods with the Nadi Technique that are simple but nonetheless extremely effective. First of all, the fact that the body is an energy source must be accepted. Let us first consider the Nadis in the hands. Shall we say that an integral part of the network of Nadis are those located in the hands; a little stimulation of these will have an incredible effect on the transportation of prana along the channels leading to the heart, the epicentre of emotional wellbeing. The treatment procedures in the Nadi Technique may not necessarily concur with the ones with which you are already familiar, simply because with these treatments we are not only dealing with the Nadis themselves, but also the more subtle channels within the Nadis. This is the reason why the Nadi treatments are so varied and really do cover a wide area of the subtle anatomy.

TAPPING TO RELEASE NEGATIVE EMOTIONS

Step 30: Release of emotions

To begin with, locate the fleshy part at the edge of the hand, on the side of the little finger.

Now, gently tap the fleshy part of the hand, four times, whilst saying out loud, "I am letting go of all my negative emotions, and now I want to be more positive and confident."

Pause for a few moments, before repeating the same process, with the affirmation.

Now, repeat the same on the other hand. Pause for a moment before repeating the process a second time. Pause for a few moments.

Now, tap four times, just below the bottom lip, saying out loud, "I know I have been insecure and lacking in confidence, I am letting go of that, to become more confident and successful in everything I undertake."

Pause for a few moments, then repeat the tapping process again, whilst saying the affirmation out loud.

Pause for a few moments, before gently tapping above the top lip, just below the tip of the nose, saying, "I am now going to be positive, dynamic and charismatic, free from all my insecurities."

Repeat the tapping in the same place, again saying the same affirmation.

Now, pause for five minutes whilst sitting quietly with your eyes closed, contemplating your life with a completely different attitude, with no insecurities and more confidence.

Now, with the right hand closed into a fist, gently tap the area of the heart, saying the affirmation, "I am no longer insecure; I am relaxed, confident and successful. I am no longer insecure; I am relaxed, confident and successful."

Pause for a few moments and repeat the whole process of tapping the heart with your fist and repeating the same affirmation.

On the conclusion of the tapping, pause for a few moments, before gently slapping your chest simultaneously with both open palms, saying the affirmation, "I have finally released all my negative energies, and am now a completely new person. I have finally released all my negative energies, and am now a completely new person."

There are many variations of the "tapping" procedures, but as long as the affirmations are repeated with a positive attitude and a forceful tone, with the belief that it is going to work, then great benefit will be derived.

It must always be borne in mind, that the body is a veritable network of Nadis, relentlessly conveying Prana from strategic locations along the surface of the subtle anatomy, to the organs of the physical body. The emotional structure of the Nadi network is located around the area of the heart, the solar plexus, and the head. An emotionally insecure person benefits greatly from tapping strategically in these areas.

Step 31: Grounding

Sit comfortably on a straight-back chair, and breathe rhythmically, making sure that the inhalations and exhalations are even spaced.

When you feel quite relaxed, focus your attention on both temples either side of your head. And with the index fingers of both hands, gently tap these areas four times, saying out loud, "I am now more focused, and emotionally grounded." Repeat this

126

affirmation four times. (Not necessarily simultaneously with the tapping.)

Repeat that process one more time, along with the affirmation.

Now, focus your attention on the area of the heart. Sit quietly contemplating the heart and feelings of love and sensitivity. Then, placing the left hand on top of the right hand, gently tap the heart with both open palms, four times, saying "I am happy, emotionally secure and filled with love and compassion." Repeat the tapping along with the affirmation once more.

Now, focus your attention on the area around the solar plexus. Sit quietly contemplating the solar plexus.

Do the same as you did with the heart, place your open left palm over the right hand, and gently tap your tummy four times, saying out loud, "I am strong, confident and can see a positive future. I now let go of all my insecurities and weaknesses." Repeat the process twice, before relaxing. Conclude the exercise with some rhythmic breathing, before drinking a glass of charged water.

The process of tapping also works at a subconscious level, and encourages the movement of Prana along the Nadis. To produce positive results, it should ideally be carried out two or three times a day. Always make sure you are totally relaxed, and that your mind is focused on the actual process of tapping.

You can either integrate the "tapping" process with other treatments in the programme, or simply use it on its own. Remember, you don't have to use the entire Nadi system; just use the methods that suit you best. You may even choose to select several of the treatments to format your own Nadi healing system. Use whatever works for you.

I have already explained that the body itself consists of a network of Nadis, along which Prana is constantly transported, in the relentless maintenance of the body's health and vitality. The Nadi Technique helps to maintain order by overhauling this delicate network, ensuring its upkeep and viability. The hands are an integral part of the Nadi network, and maybe used to assess the reliability of the flow of Prana through strategic parts of the body. Should you feel a little tenderness while gently tapping the knuckles and the backs of the hands, then this is a reliable indication that a blockage is occurring in the system as a whole.

Step 32: Assessing occurring blockage

First of all, place your left hand flat on a table, palm down with the fingers spread.

Place the tip of your ring finger of your right hand on top of the nail of your pointing finger.

Now, gently tap each knuckle of the left hand, making a note of any sensitivity, however slight. It may be necessary to repeat this tapping process a few times.

Finally, still with the ring finger touching the pointing finger, tap the back of the left hand, beginning below the little finger, and concluding below the thumb, again making a note of any sensitive, however slight.

Now, repeat the same process, gently tapping the right hand. Again making a note of any sensitivity, regardless of how slight.

Any sensitivity that you feel is indicative of minute blockages along the Nadis. Although the blockages occur in the subtle anatomy, they will eventually impact upon the corresponding parts of the physical body. Prevention is always much better than cure, as they say; and so with a little manipulation in strategic

128

spots, the blockage can easily be relieved. The Nadi Technique may not necessarily concur with the traditional knowledge you may already have of complementary treatments, as this system of addressing subtle energy problems is a little different, inasmuch as with this system of healing we are treating the subdivisions of the Nadis themselves. The human organism itself is subdivided into seven, and so on through infinity. Not only can the Nadi technique be used to treat a condition after it has occurred in the physical body, but the treatment can also be applied to predict the onset of illness or disease.

Once the area where the sensitivity has occurred has been located, simply tap it gently three or four times, and immediately follow this by vigorously rubbing the area at the same site.

Repeat the process four or five times, or until the sensitivity is no longer felt. Please do not make the mistake of dismissing the process on its simplicity. As I have explained all through the book, although the Nadi Technique is a unique self-healing system that is extremely easy to use, its effects are quite spontaneous and really do cover a very broad spectrum of treatments. Although the physical procedures of the Nadi Technique are important, and therefore are an integral part of the overall treatment, it also helps when the process is carried out with a little mental interaction. As you become familiar with the way the Nadi healing system actually works, so the more confidence you will have in it. The Nadi Technique works at an extremely subtle level and affects the physical body holistically.

Applying pressure to ease toothache and neuralgia

Remember, Nadi Technique should be used to complement traditional allopathic treatments, and not to replace them. Use this particular treatment to ease the discomfort of pain, until such time as you can seek medical attention.

When toothache strikes, or you experience the excruciating pain of neuralgia, more-often-than-not, it's in the middle of the night, when the only option is to take some pain relief, or put up with it until the morning. The following may help in the short-term.

Step 33: Relieving pain

Lay the hand that corresponds with the side of the face that is affected, flat on your lap, with the fingers and thumb spread apart.

Take the thumb of the other hand and place it firmly on the fleshy part, between the thumb and pointing (index) finger, as far into the joint as possible, with the pointing finger on the opposite side of the thumb.

Now, apply as much pressure as you can into the fleshy part between the thumb and index finger of the hand being treated, either until a slight tingling sensation is experienced on the side of the face where the pain is felt, or for a minute, whichever comes first.

Repeat the process three or four times, with a few seconds break between treatments. Repeat this process again an hour later.

Always apply the treatment on the hand corresponding with the affected side of the face.

Conclude the process by vigorously rubbing the fleshy part between the thumb and index finger of the hand that has been treated. As usual drink a full glass of charged water.

Chapter 21

Intention and focus

Thinking in a positive way when you are feeling depressed and out of sorts is extremely difficult, but not impossible. The first thing is to break the habit of expecting to feel depressed and miserable at the same time every day. Depression is insidious and is sometimes accompanied by panic attacks. People who suffer from an acute anxiety neurosis very often subconsciously control their attacks, making them habitually regular. I know this from my own experience of the way I used to have daily panic attacks. In fact, mornings were always worse for me. Because my first panic occurred at around 9am, I used to sit watching the clock, waiting for it to happen. The Nadi Technique is also about re-aligning your thoughts, and completely changing the way you have become accustomed to thinking. Intention and focus is about just that—transforming the way you perceive your life, and psychologically moving from the dark closet you have become accustomed to living in, to a much brighter and more positive, colourful environment. Although we have explored some techniques to address this in an earlier chapter, here I would like to make a detailed analysis of alternative thinking, primarily with the sole intention of taking control of your life. Routine and order, combined, is the first step to taking control. Very often, people who suffer from some sort of depressive illness have little or absolutely no routine and order in their lives, and these are prerequisites for the road to recovery. There are physical effects as well as the psychological implications of any mental disorder, and to a person suffering with an anxiety neurosis, differentiating between the physical symptoms of a panic attack and those produced by a possible stroke or heart attack are virtually impossible. Thinking that you are having a heart attack or even a stroke tends to add fear to fear, exacerbating the horrendous experience. Once all extensive medical tests have been exhausted, and you have been reassured by your medical specialist that there is nothing whatsoever organically wrong with you, then you need to take things in hand and begin your intent and focus programme.

Firstly, give honest answers to the following questions.

When you are in the grip of a panic attack, do you really and truly believe you are going to die?

Whatever feelings you experience, do they simply disappear when you are in the presence of a medically qualified practitioner?

Do you over-indulge with anything in your daily diet?

Is your depression or anxiety worse after you have had a cup of coffee, tea or any alcoholic beverage?

Is your sleep broken several times through the night, causing you to wake in the morning feeling quite exhausted?

Are you short tempered?

Does the least little thing irritate you?

Do you find it difficult to concentrate on anything for long periods?

Do you find yourself daydreaming a lot?

Do you have absolutely no interest in things of beauty?

Even if you said yes to fewer than five of the above questions, the body and mind are not synchronized; probably the result of lack of Pranic energy to the solar plexus and the Nadis feeding that area. This may very well sound a little far-fetched to you, but even so, a few exercises to address the problem cannot in anyway do any harm.

The other thing which can cause more than one problem is dehydration and an inadequate diet. It is important that you take notice of your body and listen to what it is trying to tell you. Take notice of any unusual sensations, such as cramps in any part of the body, tingling hands, headaches and even irritability. Energizing the body by drinking plenty of charged water. Keep a glass or even a bottle of water by the bed. Should you wake in the middle of the night with a dry mouth, drink some water. Before swallowing the water, wash it a few times around your mouth and gums.

An excellent and yet an extremely effective exercise, and one that should ideally be practised in the morning and last thing at night before retiring, is this:

Step 34: Rocking chair exercise

Sit on the floor and pull your knees as close to the body as you can, with your feet flat on the floor. Clasp your hands around you knees to ensure you keep them in position and also to hold yourself in place.

Now bend forward as far as you can, then roll back on your spine to the original position.

Once you have got the gist of this movement, rock your body backward and forward several times, without stopping and without straightening the spine.

Now pause for five minutes. Straighten your legs and lean back on your hands.

Now repeat the same process several more times, with more vigour than the first time, but making certain you are not causing any discomfort to occur on any part of your body.

Now relax. Conclude the exercise by drinking a glass of charged water.

Repeat the same exercise last thing at night, about an hour before retiring.

This exercise will ensure you have a restful and good night's sleep.

A lot of the time an anxiety attack can be brought on because of tension in the neck or at some location in the spine. As I have explained in an earlier chapter, if allowed to build up through the day, or even through the week, tension can cause many different sensations in the body, from dizziness, headaches and then eventually erupt into panic attack. Although the book is not about Yoga, some of the more simple yogic exercises are ideal for precipitating Prana through the network of Nadis, thus alleviating physical and mental traumas. The word Yoga means "Union"; in fact, exercises to encourage the unification of the Ha and Tha energies—the male and female aspects of the subtle nature. For this reason I have included some very simple Yogic exercises into the Nadi system of healing. This following exercise is an excellent way of easing the trauma on the spine very often caused by bad posture. The spine houses the main Nadi called Sushumna, and is therefore an extremely important conduit for the transportation of Prana throughout the body. You may wonder what these exercises have to do with the title of the chapter Intent and Focus. Intent and Focus is also about being aware of the individual components that make-up the body, ensuring that they all work in harmony together so that balance is maintained to promote good health and longevity. Once the body begins to break down with the passage of time, it's very difficult for the mind to focus in a positive way. When used correctly with positive intent, the *will* becomes a powerful force. Belief in yourself and what you are capable of is also a prerequisite in the whole process of self-discovery and the overall healing of the body and mind. Let's take a look at this next exercise.

If for some reason you find it difficult lying on the floor, then lying on the bed is acceptable.

Step 35: The arch

Lie down flat and pull your feet as close to the body as possible so that your knees brought up.

Close your eyes and place your hands by your sides to give you some leverage.

Now raise your back and bottom off the floor (or bed), and at the same time inhale a complete breath and holding it for as long as possible, whilst maintaining the arched posture.

Exhale the breath whilst lowering your back to a resting position. Pause for a few moment.

Repeat the same process, all the time with your eyes closed.

Even if you feel a little discomfort, try to persevere, as it will help to strengthen your spine and release any tension you have allowed to build up there through poor posture etc.

I have previously explained that within the spine Sushumna, one of the major Nadis is located. Sushumna is responsible for the transportation of Prana, and is met at strategic points by the other two primary Nadis, Ida and Pingala. It is paramount that Prana flows freely along all three Nadis, and any occurring congestion will result in physical as well as psychological problems. More importantly, if your lifestyle causes you to be stressed, this will impact on the Nadis, also causing the Prana to congest. The following procedure will help.

When you are tense and feeling overwhelmed with tiredness brought on by stress, a simple procedure will invigorate you and make you feel more relaxed and yet full of energy. In other words, it will instantly recharge your depleted energy resources.

Step 36: Spinal recharging

Sit on a straight back chair with the spine erect and your eyes closed.

First of all, breathe rhythmically until the rhythm is fully established, making sure that the inhalations and exhalations are evenly spaced and yet not strained

Place the thumb and first two fingers of your hand at the base of your skull, slightly left of the spinal cord, and apply a little pressure.

Next, breathe in through the nostrils, holding the breath for a few seconds before breathing out through the mouth.

Repeat the whole breathing process four or five times, and then relax your breathing, at the same time as maintaining the position of the fingers on your neck for a further four seconds.

Now relax with the palms of your hands resting on your lap, still with your eyes closed.

You should always begin and conclude your working day with this recharging exercise. The benefits are usually felt within seconds, especially when you are tense and mentally exhausted.

INTENTION AND FOCUS

As I have said in a previous chapter, stress is insidious, the effects of which creep up on you unexpectedly. When tensions is constantly allowed to build up through each day, it is extremely difficult to eradicate. If it is not dealt with, then its implications cover a very broad area of the health. It affects your skin, your hair, your overall posture, your gait and the way you think. In fact, stress affects your physical as well as your psychological health, and can eventually cause the heart to overload. Stress accounts for more deaths than any other condition. Using the Nadi Technique will enhance the overall quality of your life, allowing you to have a clearer and much healthier perspective of life.

Chapter 22

Nutrition: healthy lifestyle

Although now a much used cliché, "you are what you eat" today has nonetheless become the mantra of the self-conscious eater, especially for those who follow a yogic way of life. What you eat and how you eat affects the individual components of your body, either for the better or for the worse. I personally have been a non-meat eater from between the ages of nine and twelve, and I haven't drunk milk since I was very young. I just did not like the taste of milk and hated the way it made me feel, all clogged up and wheezy. Although my mother greatly opposed my decision not to eat meat, it was my choice and she eventually respected it. In fact, she made some superb dishes for me and an extremely tasty pea soup. Although in later years she admitted to me that she used to occasionally flavour her pea soup with a ham bone, as she thought I needed the nutrition only a meat substance could provide. Needless to say I forgave my mother as most people in her working-class generation were of the same opinion, and that is we need meat in our diet to survive. Of course this is absolutely nonsense. I've already explored the reasons for a non-meat diet in a previous chapter, so here I would welcome my wife, Dolly's input. Dolly has had many years' experience in Corporate Hospitality; organizing huge events in and around London; apart from this, she is a first class cook with an abundance of knowledge concerning the nutritional value of food and its effect upon your health. On some of my events she has cooked for as many as forty vegetarians.

Dolly's input: suggestions for your diet

The day should begin and end with a glass of water. This should not be gulped, but sipped slowly, allowing the water to remain in the mouth for a few moments before swallowing it. This allows the Prana in the water to be absorbed by the Nadis in the tongue. As it has already been explained in an earlier chapter, water should be pour from one glass to another, backwards and forwards through the air, until it almost sparkles and comes alive with vitality. This pouring process precipitates the Prana in the water, making it more potent.

Some people are only concerned about the flavour of the food they cook, giving little or no regard at all for the nutritional value. Although today the majority of people do have an interest in healthy eating, there still appears to be some ignorance about the full nutritional value of food. American surgeon, Dr George W Crile (Ohio, 1864—1943) believed that "all natural deaths (except old age) are merely the end point of progressive acid-saturation." In fact, in spite of all the available information regarding diet and nutrition, the majority of people still overload their digestive systems with potentially harmful and unwholesome foods. The majority of people tend to pay more attention to the food they give to their pets rather than the food they lay on their own tables.

Foods to avoid: Fried foods produce acreolin which irritates your stomach. Also, it's known that fried foods take longer to digest, particularly fatty meat products, such as bacon. Fat is the last to leave your stomach, carbohydrates leave first and proteins

139

second. It might sound like common sense, but never over-indulge, regardless of how tempted you are by a delicious meal. It's not the amount you eat and drink that nourishes your body, as much as it is the amount your digestive system is able to assimilate. Never throw away the water in which vegetables have been cooked, this contains all the mineral salts essential for a healthy digestive system. Always thoroughly wash your vegetables and cook them unpeeled. Drinking the juice fruit, vegetables and greens is highly nutritious.

Try to avoid eating more than one starch during your meal. The majority of people consume far too much starch in a meal. Never eat bread, potatoes, rice and macaroni in the same meal. And avoid eating gravy, soups and deserts prepared with flour, or pastry or cakes in the one meal. A lot of this is common sense, but you would be surprised how people are still quite ignorant today about what and what not to eat. Over-indulging every time you eat with very little exercise, causes weight gain, constipation, diabetes and many other health conditions affecting the stomach, kidneys and liver, not to mention the entire digestive system.

Cooked sulphur foods such as cabbage, cauliflower, peas, turnips, eggs and others, eaten together with starch will result in a lot of gas by the sulphur working on starch. It is always better to eat sulphur foods raw, or, if you suffer with a lot of wind, avoid mixing them with starchy foods. Also, whenever possible always eat the skins of fruit and whatever vegetables you can tolerate. Wash fruit and vegetables well, and never peel them.

You should always pay attention to how you eat as much as to the consideration of what food you eat. Your food should be chewed properly, particularly starchy foods. Whilst in your mouth the saliva converts starch into glucose and dextrin,

NUTRITION: HEALTHY LIFESTYLE

otherwise it ferments in the stomach for several hours. Always sip your liquids slowly instead of gulping them quickly. The longer liquid remains in your mouth, the more Prana you will absorb. Besides this, if you gulp your fluids you are likely to get indigestion. Many people who follow a strict Yogic diet, avoid eating vegetables that grow beneath the soil, such as carrots and potatoes, and eat only those that ripen in the sunlight. A light breakfast is preferable to a fully cooked one. The reason being, a heavy breakfast draws the blood from the head to the stomach, and the head cannot be light and clear while the stomach is full and heavy. Yogic practitioners always eat their last meal of the day before sunset. After that it is advisable to take only water or juices. This allows the digestive system to fully recover whilst you sleep.

There is very little doubt that our eating habits very often originate from our parents, who are responsible for what we eat and the way we eat.

A healthy approach to the day, especially if you are trying to lose a little weight, could be the following.

Try starting the day with a 6oz glass of diluted grape juice, sipped slowly before breakfast. Or, if you prefer, a glass of diluted Cranberry juice.

For breakfast, fresh raw fruit, especially citrus, with some plain yoghurt. If you don't like yoghurt, a handful of nuts could be eaten as an alternative.

An alternative suggestion could be some salad with a handful of nuts.

Midmorning: A small portion of fresh vegetables, perhaps a carrot or a couple of celery sticks and some sliced apple. You could include a few almonds with this. Instead of coffee or tea, try a cup of herbal tea, or even Dandelion coffee. Eliminate caffeine completely from you diet. Don't forget, tea also contains caffeine.

Half an hour before lunch have a glass of diluted red grape juice.

For your lunch have a raw mixed salad containing at least three vegetables that grow above the ground. This could either include some fish and or a baked potato with the skin. Don't have a baked potato more than twice a week. You could include a little Tofu with this. However, it is all a matter of taste.

The idea is to recondition your digestive system so that it does not crave for food and to stop you picking.

Don't forget the water charging process. Always pour the water through the air from one glass to another. This precipitates the water's Pranic content and makes it come alive. You will notice the difference in its taste. Remember, always sip your water and never gulp it. Allowing it to remain for a few seconds in your mouth gives the Nadis in your tongue more time to absorb and assimilate the Prana more efficiently.

Regardless of what is wrong with you, moderate exercise is essential. Even a casual walk in the park is extremely beneficial to the body, mind and spirit, and helps to lift you from depression. When you wake up in the morning, if you know you're not going to go back to sleep, get up and throw yourself into your day. Never lie there thinking about all the things that have happened to you, or the things that could happen to you. Remember what I have said in previous chapters; dwelling too much on anything can make it happen. Get into the habit of focusing in a positive way, without revisiting the past. Try saying out loud to yourself "Every day in every way I am feeling better and better and better. Every day in every way I am feeling better and better and better."

Repeat it several times whilst sitting on the edge of your bed. Use it as your morning mantra. This will help to instil your subconscious mind with new and more positive energies, and will help to clear out the negative memories in the whole process of reprogramming your mind to be more focused on a brighter, happier and healthier life.

I know from my own experiences just how difficult it is to think in a positive way when you are feeling depressed, miserable and very unhappy. It is an extremely lonely, solitary journey, but one that is necessary if you are ever to take control again of your life.

Chapter 23

Change, growth, and freedom

Freedom and Change are included within the parameters of the self-healing system of the Nadi Technique, for the whole process is about addressing the numerous psychological, emotional and physical issues that have held you back and impaired the quality of your life for so long. It's also about setting yourself free from all the hang-ups that impose so many restrictions on your life and make you unhappy. Although the principles of the Nadi Technique are not connected to any one particular religious system; they do have a common theme, and that is self-realization and personal development combined. Change must come before freedom can become a reality. I have said all through this book that we are the architects of our own destinies simply by the way we think. The personal issues you have been struggling with are really insignificant, and whether they are physical or psychological, the process and treatment are the same. More often than not an individual is influenced by the environment in which they live, as well as the pressures imposed upon them by other people. Creating the right environment does not necessarily imply the dynamic alteration of existing conditions. Sometimes it is not worth the effort required to move what is inert. The things that are affecting you in your existing environment may in fact be so great that any hope of bringing about change through your personal efforts may seem absolutely futile; or perhaps you feel that it would require more effort and time than you have in the years you have left. If such is the case, it is sometimes much wiser to retreat from the circumstances you find yourself in and begin anew elsewhere. This may seem somewhat defeatist; but after all, what you are really seeking is not a flush of victory or conquest but rather a new series of conditions or different elements of living. Bringing about dramatic changes to a lifestyle to which you have been accustomed for so long is perhaps the most difficult thing you have ever been faced with, but most certainly not impossible.

Challenge is necessary for growth and evolution in life. Without challenge, life would become stale and stagnant. But what challenges do you choose to address, those offered by society and the environment in which you live, or the ones that arise from the deepest recesses of your own soul? I know you may well think that the challenges, tensions and conflicts you are forced to face on a daily basis are presented to you from the outer and not the inner world; but the outer environment is in many ways a reflection of what is occurring within you. Remember, thoughts crystallize into habit, and habit solidifies into circumstances. Before your circumstances can ever change, you must first of all change the way you have become accustomed to thinking. Your awakening consciousness will communicate to others, and will raise in them a similar capacity. The influence of your life will emanate from you just like the scent of the flower. The rose releases its fragrance to the air impregnating everything around it with its delicate emanations. And the same phenomenon occurs with the transformations you have made to the way in which you think. They not only affect your own life, but they also affect the lives of those around you. You may initiate changes in the way you think, but if your heart cannot move on, as they say, then nothing else around you will change. Should your problem be addiction of some kind, then the way you perceive that addiction will impact upon your ability or inability to control it. If you perceive your addiction as a weakness, then the way you regard your addiction will really make it into a weakness that you will find even more difficult to overcome. Determination is very much a prerequisite for you to take control of any craving that is controlling you. You need to control it instead of allowing it to control you. You need to be the master of your own life, and encourage the heart and mind to focus on the same goal. I am writing this from my own experience; and I know only too well how addiction affects one's life and the lives of those around you. My own struggles brought me to the realization that addiction is a lonely road. I could not even see the slightest glimmer of hope on the horizon, and seriously considered ending my life. Had it not been for the comforting and yet direct words of a young psychiatrist in a clinic where I was being treated, I was in no doubt about ending my life. There is always a glimmer of hope in everyone's life; it's just that it is nearly always obscured by the distorted vision of the depression brought about by a self-created darkness. Even in our darkest moments life is still precious. The onus is always on you to aspire to be positive and more focused. Nothing in this life is permanent. One moment gives way to another, transmuting one feeling into another, and causing the distortion of depression to diminish. They do say that time is a great healer. This is only true if you are strong enough to be patient, and sufficiently courageous to try to conquer those demons that lurk somewhere deep within the darkest corners of your mind, or even your soul, whatever you choose to call it. Once you have taken the decision and moved

146

one step closer to doing this, you will find that thoughts, flashes of inspiration will seem to float to the surface of your consciousness. At this point, these inspirations, occasional flashes of wisdom, will very often present other challenges, immense obstacles that will make you think that some powerful force is pulling you further down, and that glimmer of hope you had seen flickering on the horizon of your life, seems to disappear completely. There are always setbacks in everyone's life, let alone in the life of someone fighting addiction or even depression. Never allow yourself to lose heart to think that the battle is lost. These emotional and psychological setbacks are what motive you and make you strong. Where or not you accept the existence of a soul, or even a supernatural power, is not important. The truth is, once you have taken steps to conquer the demons that lurk somewhere in the darkest recesses of your own subconscious mind, you will gradually become acquainted with a strength you have never before known. These inspirations, potential or hidden forces, call them what you will, are not the products of your imagination, or some dark forces percolating from deep within your mind, with the sole intention of trapping you and sending you once again spiralling out of control back into the depths of despair. They are the products of the seeds you have sown during your darkest moments and which have gradually culminated into a dynamic force that you really are. Freedom comes about only when this transformation of consciousness occurs, causing resonance with the universe, the ultimate force that will always conspire to lead you to that place of safety where you have for so long struggled to be.

I know all this will probably sound very metaphysical to a sceptic who may even dismiss the entire book as a result of it. But the truth is, the Nadi system of healing is a holistic process, with consideration of body, mind and spirit, the subtle and metaphysical part of our being. Various laws are always in constant operation all through our lives, and the acceptance and understanding of these laws to a certain extent sets us free. The way in which we think and conduct our life has an effect on those around us. The way we think also produces a corresponding effect on the individual components of our bodies, either encouraging good health, or causing it to become unhealthy and diseased. To some extent does our environment influence the way we think as well as the way we speak. The environment in which we live also shapes our features and much of the time makes us who and what we are. As I explained in the introduction, from a very early age we are programmed by our parents, as they were programmed by their parents before them, and so on through the family history. As well as encouraging optimum health, the Nadi Technique also explores the fundamental principles underlying the supersensual side of our life, with a look at the important parts these principles actually play in the spiritual evolution of our consciousness. The precept of any Holistic therapy is "before you can treat the part, you must first consider the whole".

Chapter 24

The brain and evolution of instinct

With such advancements having been made in the field of modern neuroscience, I think it is only right to say that little consideration is given to what is referred to as the "old reptilian brain." This is the area of the brain that is responsible for our most basic instincts. Human consciousness has evolved at such a rate that we have long since forgotten how to use the natural instincts we relied on to survive in our prehistoric state. Although before we evolved even the most rudimentary form of speech, many anthropologists believe that our prehistoric forebears mostly communicated their thoughts and feelings through expressive dance, a minority believe that some also communicated their thoughts and feeling telepathically. Whether or not the latter statement is true, the fact is, unlike the majority of animals, we humans do not use the full capacity of our brains, and very little is known about the full potential of the human mind. The evolution of our emotions appears to have occurred sometime after our prehistoric ancestors lived in caves, and our emotions are responsible for many of the wrong decisions we actually make in life. Many people allow their emotions to rule their lives, whilst others appear to keep them carefully under control. Science does not fully understand how our emotions work, and although the majority of people make every effort to control their emotions, as a powerful force, our emotions always exert a powerful control over us, regardless of what we think. In fact, the emotions function to all intents and purposes just like an electromagnetic force, and are very loosely connected to our instincts and appear to be functions of the subconscious mind. Although this may only be an intellectual construct, perhaps far removed from actuality, it still serves as a very good framework upon which we can gain a thorough understanding of the inner workings of the emotions. Being properties of the mind operating on the subconscious level, the emotions, and the instincts of which they are an integral part, are tremendously powerful in the way they govern our behaviour, and indeed the way they influence the way we feel about ourselves. To a large extent the emotions also govern the very motives that drive us to do what we end up doing in life, and ultimately, the very key to mastery of life lies in learning how to direct these energies, certainly in a positive way. The emotions and in a broader sense, the instincts, therefore need to be properly understood and appreciated as necessary sources of motive power that lead us towards our own evolution.

Limbic system

The limbic system participates in the expression of emotions and also learning and memory. However, the "old reptilian" instinctual or R-complex system is also a part of the brain's vertical polarity along with the limbic and thalamic regions of the brain. Each is an integral part of the whole and each affects the other. Therefore, it is not useful at all to postulate that the instinctual or "reptilian" brain is a primitive culprit harbouring our baser emotions which then somehow have to be overcome. The instinctual brain governs all our instincts including our emotions, and many of our autonomic functions. Instincts in themselves are valuable sources of information if we can decode their messages. But they are also extremely powerful forces, literally mapping out our destiny. Although properly channelled or directed, the expression of instinct serves to guard our physical and psychic wellbeing, and it is this guarding function which is perhaps the strongest in our instinctual behaviour. In fact, one could say that the whole purpose of the instincts, or the "old reptilian brain" are for the ultimate preservation of the physical and psychic being. It has taken aeons of time to evolve to the state we are in today, and although there is no necessity for us to use our instincts today as we did and had to when we swung from trees or lived in caves, we cannot take our instinctive faculty lightly, for it literally governs who we really are and what we are capable of accomplishing.

Blocked expression in any part of the brain can ultimately lead to physical disharmony. In fact, a blocked expression is an instinctual tendency which the intellect does not allow to manifest. For one example, instinct may tell you that you need some sleep, whilst the intellect tells you that you need to press on with the task in hand and force you to stay awake. Ultimately instinct will win and you will fall asleep while you are working. Another example is when instinct allows you to be openly attracted to someone, whilst the intellect tells you that the person is just not right for you.

It only takes a single instrument playing out of tune, to destroy the harmony expressed by the orchestra as a whole. Whether in an orchestra or the human body, the attainment of harmony demands considerable effort, patience, practice, experience and intuitive development. Good health begins by perceiving all the individual components of the body as necessary instruments in the body-orchestra, even if we do not initially understand their purpose. The more we know about each part of ourselves the easier it is to appreciate each individual part's place in the general harmonium we are seeking to establish.

Remember that the physical structures of the brain are not the Mind itself. The neurological structures and neuro-chemical activities within the brain are necessary instruments of the Mind, and are well adapted to the functioning of the Mind. As the twentieth-century psychologist Arthur Koestler put it, Mind in the brain is like a "ghost in the machine", something which intangible operates the machine, but crucially depends upon its structure and correct functioning.

The horizontal and vertical polarities of the brain refer only to the physical structure through which the Mind is functioning. The horizontal polarity refers to the fact that certain functions, such as verbalization, imaging and spatial perception, are located on opposite sides of the outer brain, whilst the vertical polarity refers to the fact that the autonomic and instinctual functions are located in the inner brainstem. The horizontal and vertical anatomical polarities are also reflected by certain enzyme and electromagnetic activities. However, once again, we must remember that these activities and polarities are simply instruments which help the Mind to manifest. Mind uses these instruments as needed. We must provide the raw materials for the maintenance of these instruments with a proper diet and correct breathing. Additional physical manipulation of the brain's various parts are neither necessary nor desirable except under extremely rare circumstances. The proper unfoldment of the brain's potential takes place naturally in accordance with the individual's ability to allow the intelligence inherent in each cell to manifest in accordance with a general body harmonium, a harmonium which is ultimately under the direction of the Mind. The keys to emotional health lie within each person. They are slowly revealed through personal experience, through reflecting upon the law of cause and effect in one's actions, and through the functioning of the human spirit which ever encourages us to wholeness. We shall attain our goals of harmony, love and peace of mind because these are the gifts of our own nature. So, you must never despair, for your path through life mirrors your own nature and sacred gifts contained within.

The various healing treatments included in the Nadi Technique also encourage emotional balance by streamlining the neurological circuitry and infusing it with the all essential life-giving prana. Meditation also helps to create a bridge of consciousness and causes an alteration in the neurological circuitry in the brains of those who meditate religiously every day. It also helps the meditator to bring his or her emotions under greater control, a necessity where the majority of people are concerned. As I have explained in an earlier chapter, scientific research carried out in California University showed conclusive evidence that the brains of those who had practised meditation for some years were marginally larger than those who did not meditate. So, it is a scientific fact, meditation encourages a great neurological capacity and also helps the release of the meditator's full potential.

Tension anywhere in the body mostly originates from the back of the neck, the spine and across the shoulders. This causes the free-flowing Prana to be restricted. A very simple exercise to release the inhibited Prana and ease tensions is one that the majority of people have done at one time or another.

Step 37: Neck and arm stretch

Sit on a straight back chair and make sure your back is as straight as possible.

Clasp both hands behind your head pushing your elbows back as far as you can.

Now, still with your hands clasped behind your head, lean as far as you can to the right. Hold it in that position for a few seconds.

Now, lean to the left as far as you can. Hold that position for a further few seconds.

Now, still with your hands clasped behind your head, push your head forward, so your chin touches your chest, but try not to strain it, and hold that position for a few seconds.

Now, still with your hands clasped behind your head, push your head back, as far as is comfortable for you, and hold that position for a few seconds.

Finally, bring your head back to the initial position and place your hands on your lap and relax.

This helps to dissipate the tension at the back of your neck and encourages the Prana to flow freely down the spine and the main Nadi Sushumna. It also encourages a relaxed and calm mind.

As with all Nadi treatments drink a glass of freshly charged water.

Chapter 25

Nadi revitalizing breath

This is an excellent exercise for revitalizing and energizing the nervous system, and is a pick-me-up when you are tired or out of sorts.

Step 38: Energizing breath
Stand erect and slowly inhale a complete breath.

Retain the breath and extend your arms straight in front of you, but do not allow any tension to occur in them.

Slowly draw the hands back to your shoulders, gradually tensing the muscles in your arms and closing your hands into fists, so that when your hands reach your shoulders your hands and arms are as rigid and tremulous as you can make them.

Now, maintaining the tension in your arms and fists, push the fists slowly out, before drawing them rapidly back, still maintaining the tension. Repeat that movement seven times.

Forcibly exhale through the mouth, then relax.

You need to read this exercise through several times until you've fully got the gist of it. You may find the breath retention a little too much when you first do the exercise, but once you've fully mastered it the breath retention should not present any problems for you.

Another extremely powerful breathing exercise is the "Vocal Exercise". This exerts an incredible amount of power on the

Nadis in the throat and neck and also helps to make the overall sound of the voice clearer and much more distinctive. It also an excellent way of treating sore throats or even cold.

This is an extremely powerful exercise that not only stimulates the Nadis, but also produces a vitalizing effect upon the nerves. It is an invigorating exercise and a tonic to the overall nervous system, and will energize you when you are feeling lethargic and out of sorts. In the initial stages this exercise must only be used occasionally.

Step 39: *The vocal breath*

Standing up straight, slowly and steadily inhale a complete breath, filling the lungs as much as you can, and taking as much time as possible.

Retain the brain for a few seconds, making sure that you are not straining it.

Now, expel the air vigorously, in one breath, open the mouth as wide as possible.

Now relax your breathing, bringing the inhalations and exhalations back to normal, but making sure that they are evenly spaced.

Practise this exercise once every couple of days, making sure that it is never a strain. You should notice a difference in the sound and tone of your voice in a very short time. It has the effect of stimulating all the Nadis in the throat and nasal areas, strengthening your vocal organs.

Yogi Masters have used breath control for thousands of years as a means of enhancing the quality of their lives, as well as encouraging altered states of consciousness. I have explained in a previous chapter that in the western world we have become accustomed to breathing incorrectly. And from a very early age we are taught to expand the chest to fill the lungs with air as we breathe-in, and close it as we breathe-out. Correct breathing must include the diaphragm in the process of breathing, and although the chest is involved in certain types of rhythmic breathing, to ensure we obtain the maximum amount of Prana from each breath, you need to ensure that you are mindful that the inhalations and exhalations are evenly spaced. The Yogis have a particular breathing exercise that I have found useful and which I have included in the Nadi Technique. They call this the "Cleansing Breath" as it ventilates and cleanses the lungs, excellent when you have been suffering with a chest infection. It stimulates the cells and gives tone to the respiratory organs, encouraging them back to good health.

Besides this, it refreshes the mind as well as the respiratory system.

Step 40: Cleansing breath

Stand up straight, inhale a completely breath.

Retain the breath for a few seconds, without straining it.

Pucker up the lips as though you are going to whistle, but make sure you do not puff-out the cheeks, then forcibly exhale a little of the breath through the lips. Pause for a moment retaining the breath.

Now forcibly exhale a little more of the air from your lungs, and then pause again for a moment.

Finally, forcibly exhale the last of the air from your lungs. Remember to purse your lips all through the exercise, and to exhale with as much force as you can.

The cleansing breath should be practised regularly until you have fully mastered it. Used when you are exhausted it will invigorate and revitalize you. Yogi Masters always conclude all their breathing exercises with the Cleansing Breath as this has the effect of sealing everything by infusing the nervous system with Prana.

Breath is life; life is solely dependent upon breath. In fact, it is during the process of respiration that Prana collects in certain bodily centres, particularly the solar plexus, from where it is constantly dispensed throughout the body. So, you should now begin to see that Prana has its own particular parts to play in the manifestation of life, apart from the physiological functions. I explained in an earlier part of the book that 60 deep breaths should be taken during the course of the day, obviously not all in succession. As well as this you should practise breath retention as often as you possibly can. It is known that frequently retaining the breath strengthens and develops the respiratory system, as well as strengthening the organs of nutrition, the nervous system and helps to make health blood. Once a complete breath has been taken, hold the breath for as long as is comfortable. Try this several times a day. As well as improving lung capacity, it also oxygenates the blood and purifies the air that has remained in the lungs from previous inhalations. It is extremely effective where there are disorders of the stomach, liver and blood. It also helps to eradicate halitosis (bad breath) by encouraging the expulsion of harmful waste in the lungs.

Step 41: Breath retention

Stand up straight, shoulders thrown back, ensuring that the spine is straight.

NADI REVITALIZING BREATH

Slowly inhale a complete breath.

Retain the breath for as long as you can, without feeling any discomfort.

Exhale vigorously through the open mouth.

If you feel you can, repeat this process once more.

Conclude this with the cleansing breath previously show.

Drink a glass of freshly charged water.

It's not necessary to practise all the breathing exercises in the book, but just select the ones you feel are beneficial for you.

An ideal exercise to begin your day is this:

Step 42: Morning exercise

Stand erect, with your shoulders back, as though standing to attention, with your head up, eyes to the front, your legs stiff and your hands by your sides.

Slowly raise your body standing on your toes, slowly and steadily inhaling a completely breath as you do.

Hold the breath for a few seconds, maintaining the same position standing on your toes.

Slowly exhale through the nostrils, lowering yourself until both feet are flat on the ground.

Repeat the same process, only this time standing on the toes of your left foot and allowing your right foot to remain flat on the ground.

Now repeat the same, this time standing on the toes of your right foot and allowing your left foot to remain flat on the ground.

This exercise sounds easier than it actually is, but the breathing and elevating yourself on your toes will require a little practice before it can be carried out correctly.

Chapter 26

Chant your way to good health

The majority of people do not realize the importance of the vibrations of sound and the effect they have on the body and mind. We know only too well how good we feel after a good old belly laugh. It invigorates us and it feels as though we've just finished exercising or working out in the gym. A good laugh encourages the release of endorphins and other enhancing chemicals in the body, and it is this physiological phenomenon that makes us feel good after a laughing fit. The vibrations of chanting also have the same effect on the body, and the varying tones of chanting produce different effects on the major glands of the body, stimulating and invigorating them. Even singing at the top of your voice in the show makes us feel good about every-thing. As I have explained in an earlier chapter, everything is in constant vibration, and within that vibration is to be found a certain rhythm. Rhythm in fact pervades the universe, and the individual components that make up the human organism also vibrate with a certain rhythm. Chanting in anyway encourages harmony within the body and the mind, and promotes balance and good health throughout our inner as well as our outer lives. If I placed two stringed instruments, perhaps guitars, in opposite corners of a room, and plucked the G string of one instrument, the G string on the other instrument would sound in sympathetic resonance. Although a simple analogy it explains perfectly well the concept of vibration and resonance between two different bodies. The Nadi Technique is also about creating harmony in your body and in everything else around you. By sounding all the existing vowels using the power of the breath, is it then possible to improve the overall health. It certainly lifts the spirits when you are feeling out of sorts or even depressed. The vibrations of sound can be so powerful as to break glass or even cause a landslide to occur. Soldiers marching in time across a bridge are given the command to break their step, simply because the constant vibration and rhythm of the synchronized marching has the power to destroy the bridge. The repetitious intonation vowels can in time restore the health of body and mind. In Yoga chanting is a threefold practice, affecting body, mind and spirit. As long as a complete breath is used, the whole process of chanting is extremely soothing, and affects the entire system, our nerves, glands and brain.

Before I go into the process of chanting more deeply, try the following exercise just to give you some idea of how it feels.

First of all, inhale a complete and deep breath: then with the full force of your breath, sound a vibrant EEEEEEE (as in *sheep*), with your lips parted as though you were smiling. The sound you make should be consistent from beginning to the end, and should be concluded leaving a little air left in your lungs. The same pitch should be maintained all through the chanting. Remember, on the conclusion of your chanting to make certain there is a little air left in your lungs, as this makes it less of a labour. This is just one example of chanting, and there are of course other sounds to influence different parts of the anatomy. Let us now take a closer look at the different vowels and how they can be used in the process of healing the body and the mind.

Step 43: The full potential of chanting

EE (as in *bee*): Sounding this like a bee vibrates in the brain, affecting the pituitary and pineal glands, and the whole neurological circuitry.

E (as in *bed*): This affects the throat, larynx, tracheas, the thyroid and parathyroid glands.

A (as in *bat*): This benefits the upper respiratory system and helps to ease congestion.

AW (as in *bawl*): This has a remarkable effect on the middle of the chest, encouraging greater lung capacity.

O (as in *bone*): This affects the lower part of the respiratory system, as well as the heart, liver and stomach.

OO (as in *boot*): This affects the kidneys.

OO-EE (as in *gooey*): This affects the bowel, rectum and the gonads of the male and female reproductory system.

An excellent and extremely effective sound for vibrating the heart and surrounding areas is one that I occasional use, especially if I am feeling a little sorry for myself. Although it is effective with some startling results, it should only be used once a day, and avoided altogether if you suffer with heart problems.

Inhale a completely breath, then as vigorously as possible, sound

MMMMMMM-PO-MMMMMMM

Remember to use the full force of your breath, this time maintaining the sound until all the air has been fully expelled from your lungs. On the conclusion of sounding this, sit quietly for a few minutes. Finish off with a glass of charged water. Never gulp the water, but always sip it slowly, washing it around your

162

mouth for a few seconds giving the Nadis in the tongue a chance to absorb the Prana in the water.

Whenever possible, practise your chanting outdoors, perhaps in the garden, weather permitting. Primarily because of the acoustics, some practitioners prefer to do their chanting in the bathroom. Vibrating the organs with the use of various sounds will help to eliminate many of our illnesses, and will also encourage a healthier body and mind.

A healthy endocrine system is the key to a long life. The vibrations of chanting stimulate the individual glands, energizing them and encouraging Pranic activity that lies dormant in them. Let's take a look at the endocrine glands and their function in the process of maintaining the health of the body.

As I explained in chapter seventeen, endocrine glands are sometimes referred to as ductless, obviously because they have no ducts and secrete their hormones directly into the bloodstream. Together they form the endocrine system, each gland working relentlessly with the other. This system is comprised of the pituitary and pineal glands situated in the cavity of the skull. The thyroid and parathyroid are located near the larynx at the base of the neck, and the thymus is located in the chest above the heart. The pair of adrenals or suprarenals top the kidneys, looking to all intents and purposes like two hoods, and then finally the gonads of the male and female reproductive system. All these glands support each other, and the working of one depends on the others. Combined it is a piece of glandular machinery that works relentlessly in maintaining the overall health of the body. Our health is solely dependent on the endocrine system's normal functions and development. The different sounds we make in the process of chanting helps to maintain balance in the endocrine system, encouraging its good health and ensuring that it is constantly enriched with vitality. This has a holistic effect upon our lives, keeping us healthy and making us feel good about ourselves and about the life around us. As one would expect, The Nadi Technique works on many different levels, from the physical level, to the more subtle areas of our life. The more you work with subtle energies, the more clearly you will begin to perceive things. An understanding of the finer and more subtle aspects of your life, will enhance the quality of how you perceive things and other people. In other words, the Nadi Technique transforms the way you think as much as it heals the body.

Overview

There is no necessity to follow the Nadi Techniques treatments chronologically as some of them may not be appropriate for you. This is a book that you can dip into when you are looking for a treatment for a specific condition. You will greatly benefit from regular use of the meditation and deep relaxation exercises, as these will enrich and improve the quality of your life on all levels. The breathing methods may be used on a regular basis, primarily to improve lung capacity and energize your body and mind. You would be advised to read through the book a few times until you fully understand what the Nadi Technique is exactly and how best to use it. Depending on the severity of your condition, the right treatment can be spontaneous with effects that are far reaching. Frequently used, some of the Nadi treatments may be used as a sort of tonic to encourage your vitality and overall performance. The Nadi Technique energizes the body to encourage optimum vitality and health. It must also be borne in mind that the Nadi Technique is a system of complementary

164

treatments and must only be used to support the treatment you may already be receiving from your medical practitioner and not to replace it. Unless, of course you are suffering with a minor condition that does not require medical treatment; in which case you can experiment with the treatments you think may well be appropriate.

In many cases of illness, the mind plays an extremely integral part, most certainly where stress and anxiety are concerned. The Nadi Technique contains various treatments to encourage a more relaxed and serene mind, with experiments to show you exactly how stressed you are. Although I have explored a non-meat diet in an earlier chapter, this is not absolutely necessary and may not appeal to you any way, particularly if you have spent a lifetime eating meat. Nonetheless, it's never too late to give a non-meat diet a try. As long as you consult your doctor before cutting out meat altogether, who knows, you may well even enjoy it.

Although I created the Nadi Technique during the 1980s, I had used many of the treatments on myself with some degree of success during the 1970s. My mother had been a great influence on my interest in complementary medicine. In fact, because of my chronic lung condition, as a child my mother frequently took me to see an old herbalist women who lived in a cottage in the middle of a wood in Wales. As we entered the woman's dimly-lit cottage I can recall being overwhelmed with an unusual pungent aroma, and the shelves around the room were filled with glass jars containing all sorts of different coloured liquids. Although we had visited the old woman on numerous occasions, she always eyed me curiously as though she was seeing me for the first time. She would sit me down, lay her hands heavily on my head, before

165

moving them slowly to my shoulders and then to my back. Before we left she would pour a small amount of red liquid from one of the jars into a glass and watch with a smile across her thin lips as I quickly swallowed it, grimacing with the taste. We would always leave with a small brown bottle containing the same liquid. I can recall my mother almost being in awe of the old woman, whose reputation as a healing "witch" was widely known throughout the little village of Gronant, north Wales. My mother later told me that she never took any payment for what she did, something I could not quite understand. The old lady always intrigued me, and although we never knew what was in her strange concoction, my mother swore by it and was quite adamant that it really did help to make me better. I suppose even at that very early age the old herbalist woman inspired me to do what I do today. Sometime during the mid-1970s I had regular visits from a healer who was sent by the National Federation of Spiritual Healers. Desmond Tierney was an exceptional man and someone who possessed a great deal of knowledge about spiritual matters. Because I had been so traumatized with my use of narcotics, he treated me with hypnosis at least once a week. Although I knew about hypnosis this was my very first experience of it as a complementary treatment. Even though I could not understand exactly how it worked, it fascinated me so much that I began to read as much as I could about it. More than all this, Desmond Tierney obviously saw that I had potential, as he gave me numerous books to read on the subject. Gradually I was developing a deep interest in healing and the art of suggestion. I had been psychic since I was a child, something I had inherited from my mother, and her mother before her. This was just something I was and not something that was an option to make a living from. Nonetheless, I was gradually becoming more and more intrigued with the subject and could not get enough of it. I spent at least an hour of each night meditating and going through my Pranayamic breathing programme. At that point I had no idea what I was trying to achieve or for that matter where it would all take me. It wasn't until I established the Thought Workshop, one of the UK's first centres for psychic and spiritual studies and alternative therapies that I seriously began to create the Nadi Technique as it is today. The more I used it the more I added to it. Although the majority of those interested in complementary treatments are more familiar with Meridians than they are Nadis, Nadis were more significant in the self-healing process I was using. The network of Nadis that permeate the body play an integral part in supporting the Meridians in the transportation of Prana throughout the body in the relentless process of maintaining the health. As I have already explained, there is no need to use all the treatments in the Nadi system chronologically, as some of them will probably not be appropriate. Some of the more specialized treatments can also be used on animals and children, proving that they are far more than psychological placebos. For example, the colour therapy treatments are safe to use and extremely effective. The chakra rotational treatments can also be used on your pets and children with some degree of success. So too can the aura cleansing treatments. Each of the Nadi Technique treatments is complete in itself. With a little experimentation you may feel it would be more beneficial if you were to modify some of the treatments and integrate them into a system you have created of your own. As the Nadi Technique covers an incredibly broad area of treatments, I am discovering new healing methods to integrate into the system all the time, and so it is changing all the time. If you are a holistic practitioner allow the Nadi Technique to inspire and motivate you. I have no doubt whatsoever that in time the Nadi Technique will transform the way you perceive holistic treatments altogether and take you to a completely different place in the field of Complementary treatments. It is a unique system of holistic healing inasmuch as it helps to transform everything about you as a person. It not only heals the physical body and the mind, but it also encourage a deeper realization of the supersensual or spiritual aspects of your life. There are occasions when you may find that "Acceptance" is the greatest of all healers, at least until you have ascertained how to initiate the appropriate changes to help you overcome either a health condition or even a problematic situation. I use the analogy here of King Canute; he tried to command the in-flowing tide to hold back! Of course, he quickly found out that he did not have the power to do that. The only way to conquer nature is by obedience. Once you comply with this universal law you can then choose from the boundless store of nature the forces that serve your purpose. By accepting an adverse condition, especially the ones created by the internal laws that govern the overall health of your body, you then see that by working with the condition instead of working against it, you are then able to bring it under your control.

Miscellaneous facts about star signs and the health

Although strictly speaking star signs do not have anything whatsoever to do with the Nadi Technique, there is some correlation between your astrological sign and your health. During my work over the years I have made some very interesting observations concerning the health. I have concluded that there seems to be some significant connection between the health conditions with which the majority of people suffer and the planetary influences at the time they were born. This may well sound bizarre, especially if you are a sceptic or medically qualified. But I have found that people born under the same astrological signs have a propensity towards the same health conditions. Remember, this is just an observation I have made over the years and not a scientific or medical fact. Although some people are exceptions to the rule, I have found that eight out of ten people under the same astrological sign will either suffer from the same health conditions or show a propensity them. Also, I have found that some signs tend to have more of a predisposition towards addiction than others. Let's take a look at some of my observations.

Element Water

Whilst those born under the signs of Cancer and Scorpio do have a tendency towards addiction, whether it be alcohol, drugs or even sex, those born under the sign of Cancer do tend to be far more emotional and inclined to allow such addictions to take control over them instead of the other way round. On the other hand, those born under the astrological sign of Scorpio are highly strung and do become addicted to substances very easily and quickly. Both Scorpio and Cancer people are prone to nervousness and frequently suffer with panic attacks and stress. Cancer people are extremely sensitive and very often suffer with stomach conditions and digestive problems. The lungs too are frequently a problem. Scorpio people are very often prone to problems with the head, such as migraines and depression.

Although the third water sign, Pisces does very often have a tendency towards addiction, they nearly always possess the ability to control it. Those born under the astrological sign of Pisces do frequently suffer with their nerves and depression. They can sometimes have a weakness in the chest, and in many cases suffer with asthma or bronchitis.

Element Fire

Those born under the astrological sign of Aries are probably one of the physically strongest of all signs. As a result of their strength, they tend not to allow themselves to give in to minor health conditions that would bother other signs, such as colds or flu. They do suffer a lot with head and spinal weaknesses, and in their mid-forties nearly always suffer with arthritic or other inflammatory conditions. A high percentage of Aries women suffer with some sort of thyroid problems or diabetes.

Those born under the astrological sign of Leo tend to suffer with minor throat infections, sinus problems and stress related illnesses. In later life they are prone to water retention problems, lower back pain and sciatica. Urinary problems also seem to present a problem in both men and women.

Those born under the astrological sign of Sagittarius tend to live of their boundless reserve of nervous energy, and as result burn themselves out very quickly. In many cases they do tend to suffer with acute anxiety neuroses, dietary problems and diabetes. Everything goes straight to their stomach, even excessive weight.

Element Earth

Those born under the astrological sign of Capricorn nearly always tend to soldier on, so to speak. A high majority of

Capricorn people, male and female, like to overindulge, and put on weight during middle age. Capricorn people worry in silence and nearly always suffer with depression and melancholy. In the cold and damp months of the winter they nearly always suffer with arthritic problems and because of low immunity generally get run down. Swollen ankles and feet can be a problem, especially if their work involves standing up all day.

Those born under the astrological sign of Taurus tend to be extremely impatient. They worry and become anxious over the most trivial things. With those born under the sign of Taurus everything is extreme, even weight gain. They are either too thin or put on too much weight. They panic very easily but rarely suffer from addictive natures. Any weight gain has an effect on the spine and lower extremities.

The Virgo person's meticulously pedantic nature very often develops into an obsession. In fact, many of those born under this sign suffer from an Obsessive Compulsive Disorder (OCD) and frequently suffer from depression. Although quite psychologically strong, it is a strength that nearly always works against them, occasionally causing him or her to find relief in either alcohol or even drugs. The positive Virgo is extremely well-balanced with only a few hang-ups.

Element Air

Those born under the astrological sign of Libra are not only extremely indecisive when faced with a decision, they are also great worriers; they either enjoy extremely good health all through their lives, or poor health most of it. However, they do tend to ignore the signs that they do have a health issue, allowing whatever is wrong to become worse. Although they appear quite strong, they can be quite emotionally and sometimes psychologically unstable. The female of the sign often suffers with gynaecological problems, the male kidney or other urinary problems.

Although those born under the Astrological sign of Aquarius do have hidden strengths, they can suffer with lung and stomach problems. They also have to take care of their diet and their propensity towards overindulging with things that please their senses. Although they will never accept it, they can possess many hang-ups, addiction being one of them. They frequently have problems with their ears, throat and nose, and are sensitive to atmospheric pollutants.

Gemini people nearly always suffer with their nerves at some point in their lives, and can be quite neurotic. The worst of those born under the astrological sign of Gemini can have a panic attack with sounding of a car horn, the most positive one will just grin and bear an extreme shock but cry about it when they alone. Gemini people talk a lot when they are nervous, and are prone to periods of just not wanting to talk to anyone, primarily to hide their sadness or grief.

As I explained earlier, some people are exceptions to this rule, and the assessments I have made here, although pretty general, are as I have observed over the past 35 years or so with people I have treated. There are, of course, innumerable other conditions, but the ones I have listed here are the ones that have responded well to the Nadi Technique treatments.

Remember too, when addressing your own hang-ups, phobias and addictions, regardless of how serious you think they are, honesty is the very best policy. The healing process can only begin to work when you admit to yourself that you do have a problem. Although this is more the case with addictions, it really does apply to all other conditions. It is my belief that within you there is more, and the whole self-help process can be spontaneous, as long as, that is, you believe that it can and will work. The various treatments in this book have been set out in such a way as to allow you to experiment to find out which ones work for you. As I have stated in an earlier chapter, you do not have to use the whole self-healing system of the Nadi Technique, as some of the treatment will not be suitable for your condition, whatever that is.

I wish you well in your use of the Nadi Technique, and hope you achieve a much healthier life, mentally and physically.

www.ingramcontent.com/pod-product-compliance
Lightning Source LLC
Chambersburg PA
CBHW031200270326
41931CB00006B/346